A Brief and Easy Introduction to

Neuroanatomy

10 Simple Chapters to Get You Started

& 150 MCQs for Quick Review

By

Magnus Bergman, MD

Disclaimer: This book is meant to be an aid to students, not a complete textbook, and by no means a source for recommendations of treatments or other actions. While the author has worked hard to find and eliminate errors, he can leave no guarantees about the accuracy of the information, and the reader must confirm all facts with other sources. The responsibility for the consequences of medical decision-making lies solely on the practitioner (and not on the author).

Welcome to this introduction to neuroanatomy!

As the title suggests, this is not a complete textbook in neuroanatomy, but a brief and accessible overview that will give you a head start before diving into the larger books.

The topic of neuroanatomy is vast and overwhelming at first, but if someone guides you through some of the fundamental concepts and major points, you will easily master the basics and create a solid foundation of knowledge, and having done that, approaching the larger books and placing every new detail in its proper place will be easier.

This doesn't mean that a brief read-through will be enough to achieve that solid foundation. As with anatomy in general, one must read and read again, often return to the books, attend lectures and preferably have the opportunity to study the subject with actual organs. Studying neuroanatomy will be frustrating, and you will occasionally lose yourself in the details. This book should be something to return to when you feel lost, to remind yourself of what the map of the landscape looks like, so that you may return to your excursions with greater confidence.

The second half of the book consists of 150 multiple choice questions, carefully designed to help you remember and connect major points and basic facts. These questions are also suitable for quick review and when preparing for tests.

While I have tried to write clearly and avoid errors, no one is perfect and mistakes occasionally show up. If you notice an error or if something seems to be weird or missing, I will be very grateful if you contact me and let me know. You will find my e-mail address in the section for sources.

It should also be noted that it is sometimes the case that different sources use different names for the same anatomical structure, or the same names for different anatomical structures. I have tried to use names for which there seems to be a consensus among at least two reliable sources, but you need to know that every once in a while, there will be a terminological mismatch. My best advice is to use the names that your professors teach you or those that are found in your assigned literature.

I have chosen to not include images in this book, and this has two reasons. First, it is assumed that you will already have a proper anatomy book with many images, and adding a handful more just for the sake of it would not be of much use. Second, I wanted this book to be brief, and if I should include images in a meaningful way, the size of the book would be too large. However, I have created an e-book with 50 selected and fully annotated images from classic anatomy books and other sources, and added 100 image-based multiple choice questions to help you learn this subject. It is called *Neuroanatomy Images: 50 Annotated Anatomical Images & 100 Image-based MCQs for Quick Review*, and is available from Amazon.

Good luck with your studies!
Magnus Bergman, MD

Table of Contents

Chapter 1

Common and Important Terminology

One of the difficult parts of learning neuroanatomy is getting familiar and comfortable with the terminology. While many terms are used in the same way as in the anatomy of the rest of the body, there are terms that are exclusive to neuroanatomy. Certain terms are also used in a slightly different way. This first chapter intends to define some of these terms, so that the following discussions will make sense; it will also make your future studies easier. Don't worry if it feels overwhelming at first - as you continue to read and use the terms, they will eventually fall into place and feel natural.

Brief overview: Cerebrum, diencephalon, cerebellum, brainstem and spinal cord

These structures constitute the **central nervous system**. The **peripheral nervous system** is the term used to describe all the nerves and other nervous structures outside of these.

The **cerebrum** is the most conspicuous part of the central nervous system and probably what most people think of as "the brain." It is divided into two similar **hemispheres** (left and right) that each has **four lobes**. It also contains deeper structures such as the **basal ganglia**.

The **diencephalon** is a structure that is surrounded by the cerebral hemispheres, and lies deep within them and on top of the mesencephalon. It includes the **thalamus** and **hypothalamus**, although some sources also list epithalamus and subthalamus as belonging to it.

The **cerebellum** means "little brain," and is the structure that is situated below the cerebrum and behind the brain stem. Like the cerebrum, it is divided into left and right **hemispheres**.

The **brainstem** is the name applied to three structures - the **mesencephalon**, the **pons**, and the **medulla oblongata** - that connect the cerebrum and diencephalon with the spinal cord. They have important functions on their own, and are not just passive structures that nerves going to and from the cerebrum pass through.

The **mesencephalon** (also known as the **midbrain**) sits below the diencephalon and above the pons.

The **pons** (meaning "bridge") sits between the mesencephalon and the medulla oblongata.

The **medulla oblongata** is a continuation of the spinal cord, which is reflected in its name; the spinal cord is called medulla spinalis in Latin, and "oblongata" means "elongated."

The **spinal cord** runs inside the vertebral column approximately from the foramen magnum of the cranium down to the first of the lumbar vertebrae. The spinal cord contains nerves that run to and from the brain, as well as so-called interneurons that modulate nerve transmission.

Terms: Supratentorial and infratentorial

These terms refer to two compartments inside the cranium, that are separated by the **cerebellar tentorium** (tentorium cerebelli), which is a continuation of the **dura mater** (see the chapter about the cranium and meninges) that extends between the **cerebellum** and the **occipital lobes** of the cerebrum.

The **supratentorial** compartment thus houses the **cerebrum** (the two large cerebral hemispheres), and the **infratentorial** compartment houses the **cerebellum** (the brain stem is sometimes also included).

Terms: Anterior and posterior

When something is described as anterior, it indicates that it is at the front of the body (or closer to the front in relation to another structure), and when something is described as posterior, it indicates that it is at the back of the body (or closer to the back in relation to another structure).

The forehead, nose, nipples and navel are all positioned on the anterior side of the body.

The big toe is obviously anterior to the heel, but the base of the big toe is still considered posterior in relation to the nail of the big toe.

Terms: Rostral and caudal

"Rostrum" is Latin for "beak," and "cauda" is Latin for "tail." Thus, rostral means "toward the beak (nose)" and caudal means "toward the tail."

If you are at a point in the middle of the spinal cord and move in the direction of the head, you are moving rostrally, and if you move in the direction of the feet, you are moving caudally. (In this situation, "cranially" is sometimes used instead of "rostrally.")

If you are at a point in the back of the head and move to the front, you are also moving rostrally, and if you go back again, you are moving caudally.

However, it should be noted that not all sources accept that "caudal" can mean "toward the back of the brain" in human anatomy, and it is good to be aware of this (they usually advocate using "posterior").

This might make more sense if you imitate a four-legged animal and stand on all fours with your face pointing forward - rostral and caudal will then be in the same direction throughout the central nervous system.

Terms: Dorsal and ventral

If you are standing up, the back of your torso is referred to as the dorsal side, and the front of your torso is referred to as the ventral side.

Likewise, the part of your spinal cord that is facing your back is referred to as its dorsal side, and the part facing your frontal side is referred to as its ventral side.

Perhaps counterintuitively, the back of your brain is not the dorsal side. Instead, the upper (superior) side of the brain is the dorsal side. Likewise, the bottom (inferior) side of the brain is the ventral side.

Again, this might make more sense if you imitate the four-legged animal with your face pointing forward (or, if you prefer standing, bend your head backwards and turn your nose toward the ceiling; now all your dorsal surfaces point to the wall behind you).

Note that these terms are almost but not completely identical to anterior and posterior. However, in areas where they are identical, they are sometimes used interchangeably, such as when the horns of the grey matter in the spinal cord are called ventral and dorsal horns in some sources, and anterior and posterior horns in others.

Terms: Medial and lateral

These terms require that you imagine a **midline** through your body (think of it as a line that connects your nose with your navel, or just think of the spinal column).

If you are describing two points somewhere on the body, the one closest to the midline is the medial point, and the one farthest from the midline is the lateral point.

As with the other terms already mentioned, a point that is medial in one situation may be a lateral point in another.

Suppose that you draw three points in a horizontal sequence to the right of your navel, and name them 1, 2 and 3, with 1 being the closest to the navel. Compared to number 1, 2 is lateral, but compared to number 3, 2 is medial.

Most of these terms can be combined in order to describe parts of an organ or the location of something with increasing precision. For example, in the frontal lobe, one can talk about both the **ventromedial** and the **dorsolateral** prefrontal cortex. You should be able to figure out how these two areas are positioned in relation to each other.

Terms: Contralateral and ipsilateral

Contralateral indicates that something is on the opposite side, and **ipsilateral** indicates that something is on the same side.

For example, damage to one side of the **cerebrum** typically causes symptoms in the **contralateral** (other) side of the body, whereas damage to one side of the **cerebellum** typically causes symptoms in the **ipsilateral** (same) side of the body.

Terms: Afferent and efferent

These terms are most often used to describe the signals coming in to or out from the nervous system.

A signal that is coming in to the nervous system - for example, a pain signal from the hand or a visual stimulus from the eye - is called **afferent**.

A signal that is coming out from the nervous system - for example, a signal that causes the hand to move - is called **efferent**.

When you test the patellar reflex (knee reflex), the first signal (from the knee to the spinal cord) is afferent, and the second signal (from the spinal cord to the knee) is efferent.

Terms: Sagittal, coronal and axial

A brain is usually sectioned, or visualized with radiologic imaging, in one of three planes - sagittal, coronal and axial (sometimes called transversal or horizontal).

A **sagittal** section is a front-to-back section through the midline of the body. It would be a section that went from the top of the head through the nose, spinal cord and navel, and end at the level where the legs start, that resulted in two halves (left and right). (A similar section that went to the left or right of the midline would be called **parasagittal**.)

The four possible directions in a sagittal section will be anterior, posterior, superior and inferior.

A **coronal** section is like a sagittal section turned 90 degrees. It would thus start at the top of the head, go through both ears and both shoulders and continue all the way down to the soles of the feet. This would also produce two halves, but in a different way - an anterior and a posterior half.

The four possible directions in a coronal section will be superior, inferior, medial and lateral.

One way to remember what an **axial** section is, is to think of the section produced by the **axe** when an executioner beheaded a person in the old days. The alternate name, horizontal, also gives a good description.

The four possible directions in an axial section will be anterior, posterior, medial and lateral.

Terms: Nuclei and ganglia

Both these terms refer to collections of neuronal **cell bodies**.

These collections are called **nuclei** (one nucleus, many nuclei) when they are found within the **central nervous system**, and **ganglia** (one ganglion, many ganglia) when they are found in the **peripheral nervous system**.

One important **exception** is the **basal ganglia**, that are found in the **central nervous system**.

Terms: Gyri and sulci

A **gyrus** is a ridge or an elevation (its plural form is **gyri**), and the surface of the cerebral hemispheres has many gyri, several of which have specific names.

The cerebellum has its own variant of ridges, which are smaller and called **folia**.

A **sulcus** is a dip or a valley (its plural form is **sulci**), and again, the surface of the cerebral hemispheres has many sulci.

A **fissure** is a deeper kind of sulcus.

Terms used mainly in embryology

The development of the nervous system during the embryonic period is a large, detailed and difficult chapter. Here, we will only brush on the surface and mention some of the biggest milestones and a couple of central facts.

In the early embryo, three **germ layers** are formed - **ecto-**

derm, **mesoderm** and **endoderm**.

The **nervous system** originates from the **ectoderm** through the **neural tube**.
The neural tube will have a rostral (cranial) and a caudal pole.

The **caudal** pole will develop into the **spinal cord**, while the more **rostral** parts will, through a series of transformations, develop into the rest of the **central nervous system**.

Rostrally, the neural tube develops **three swellings or vesicles**, called (in caudal to rostral order) **rhombencephalon**, **mesencephalon** and **prosencephalon**; these are also known as **hindbrain**, **midbrain** and **forebrain**, respectively.

These three vesicles develop further into five vesicles:

1: Prosencephalon becomes **telencephalon** and **diencephalon**.

2: Mesencephalon does not change its name and remains **mesencephalon**.

3: Rhombencephalon becomes **metencephalon** and **myelencephalon**.

The fates of these five vesicles are as follows:

1: The telencephalon develops into the cerebral hemispheres and associated structures.

2: The diencephalon develops into the mature diencephalon (thalamus and hypothalamus, mainly).

3: The mesencephalon develops into the mature mesen-cephalon.

4: The metencephalon develops into the pons and the cerebellum.

5: The myelencephalon develops into the medulla oblon-gata.

Knowing this embryological development will facilitate understanding of the anatomy of the ventricular system.

Chapter 2

Cranium and Meninges

This chapter will describe the cranium that surrounds the brain, as well as the meninges, which are structures within the cranium that also surround the brain.

Cranium

The cranium can be divided into two main parts, the **neurocranium** and the **viscerocranium**.

The neurocranium surrounds the brain, while the viscerocranium is the skeletal structure that builds up the face. We will only concern ourselves with the neurocranium here.

Bones

The neurocranium is built up by eight bones - two paired and four unpaired bones:

Frontal bone (1)
Parietal bones (2)
Occipital bone (1)
Temporal bones (2)
Sphenoid bone (1)
Ethmoid bone (1)

Sutures

The bones of the neurocranium are connected with **sutures**. Most of them are logically named after the bones that they are connecting, such as the sphenofrontal suture, but the larger sutures have special names.

Coronal suture - this is the suture that connects the frontal bone with the parietal bones; it begins and ends where the frontal and parietal bones meet the sphenoid bone. (Note that its course corresponds to the way a coronal section would run.)

Lambdoid suture - this is the suture that connects the occipital bone with the parietal bones; it begins and ends where the occipital and parietal bones meet the temporal bones.

Sagittal suture - this is the suture that connects the two parietal bones; it marks the midline of the cranial vault and runs perpendicular to and between the coronal and lambdoid sutures. (Note that its course corresponds to the way a sagittal section would run.)

The point where the coronal and sagittal sutures meet is called **bregma**, and the point where the lambdoid and sagittal sutures meet is called **lambda**.

Squamosal sutures - these are the sutures that connect

the parietal bones with the temporal bones (there is one suture on each side).

Cranial base - fossae

In the base of the skull, three fossae (bowl-like concavities) are apparent - anterior, middle and posterior.

The **anterior cranial fossa** houses the frontal lobes of the cerebrum, and is formed by parts of the frontal, sphenoid and ethmoid bones.

The **middle cranial fossa** houses the temporal lobes of the cerebrum, and is formed by parts of the sphenoid and temporal bones.

The **posterior cranial fossa** houses the cerebellum and portions of the brain stem, and is formed by parts of the occipital and temporal bones. Note that the occipital lobes of the cerebrum are not housed by the posterior cranial fossa (they sit on top of the tentorium cerebelli).

Cranial base - foramina and other openings

Many structures need to go in or out of the cranium, and they do this by entering or exiting through one of the cranium's many openings, many of which are called foramina (one foramen, many foramina). The largest and most important foramina, along with the structures that pass through them, will be listed.

The largest opening is in the center of the cranial base, in the occipital bone, and it is called the **foramen magnum** (Latin for great hole). Several structures pass through this opening, the most important being the **spinal cord**, the two **vertebral arteries**, the **anterior** and **posterior spinal**

arteries, and the spinal portions of the **accessory nerves** (cranial nerve XI).

If the foramen magnum is seen as a clock face with the anterior midpoint being 12 o'clock and the posterior midpoint being 6 o'clock, then at around 10 and 2 o'clock you will see two small openings in the occipital bone. These are the **hypoglossal canals**, through which the **hypoglossal nerves** pass (cranial nerve XII).

If you continue in roughly the same direction, there is a larger opening created where the occipital bone meets the temporal bone. This opening is called the **jugular foramen**, through which the **internal jugular vein** and three cranial nerves (**glossopharyngeal**, **vagus** and **accessory nerves**, cranial nerves IX, X and XI, respectively) pass.

Roughly anterior to the jugular foramen is the **internal auditory meatus**, housing the **facial** and **vestibulocochlear** nerves (cranial nerves VII and VIII, respectively).

If you, however, are viewing the cranium from below, there is another opening anterior to the jugular foramen. This is the **carotid canal**, which is the point of entrance for the **internal carotid artery**.

Viewing the cranial base from the inside again, there are three foramina on each side of the sella turcica (see below), in an oblique row, running in anteromedial to posterolateral direction.

The most anterior and medial of these is the **foramen rotundum**, through which the second (**maxillary**) branch of the **trigeminal nerve** passes (cranial nerve V, branch V2).

Slightly posterior and lateral to the foramen rotundum is

the **foramen ovale**, through which the third (**mandibular**) branch of the **trigeminal nerve** passes (cranial nerve V, branch V3).

Finally, posterior and lateral to the foramen ovale is the **foramen spinosum**, through which the **middle meningeal artery** passes.

Medial to the foramen spinosum is an opening that is not always seen, and that in adults is covered by cartilage. This opening is called **foramen lacerum**.

Anterior to the foramen rotundum is a rather large opening - it is so large that it no longer is called a foramen, but a fissure. Through this structure, called the **superior orbital fissure**, run (partly or completely) the **oculomotor**, **trochlear**, **abducens** and **ophthalmic** nerves (cranial nerves III, IV, VI and V1, respectively; "V1" implies that the ophthalmic nerve is the first branch of the trigeminal nerve, which is cranial nerve V), as well as divisions of the **ophthalmic vein.**

And lastly, medial to the superior orbital fissure and anterior to the sella turcica we find the **optic canals**, through which the **optic nerves** (cranial nerve II) and the **ophthalmic arteries** pass.

A selection of some other anatomical structures of the cranium not yet listed

If you look down upon the cranial base, you will note that the anterior portion of the foramen magnum is continuous with a slope, going upward and anterior. This slope is called **clivus**. Its shape allows the pons to bulge forward.

If you continue upwards and anterior beyond the clivus,

you will come across a structure called the **sella turcica**. This structure resembles a saddle (the term is Latin for Turkish saddle), and its central depression is the **hypophyseal fossa**, where the **hypophysis** (also known as the **pituitary gland**) rests.

If you continue in the anterior direction, there are two conspicuous features arising from the **ethmoid bone** in the middle of the anterior cranial fossa, called the **crista galli** and **cribriform plate** (lamina cribrosa). The crista galli (meaning comb of the rooster) shoots up and is an attachment point for the falx cerebri (see below). The cribriform plate lies below the crista galli, and is a part of the roof of the nasal cavity; it has several **olfactory foramina** through which olfactory nerves may pass.

If you instead move all the way to back of the cranium, there is a small inward projection centrally in the occipital bone, known as the **internal occipital protuberance** (protuberantia occipitalis interna). There is a corresponding projection on the outside as well, called the **external occipital protuberance** (protuberantia occipitalis externa); this can be palpated through the skin on most people.

The meninges

The meninges are three membranes that cover the structures of the central nervous system. They have a protective function, but also aid in separating the brain into compartments, as well as facilitating the circulation of blood and cerebrospinal fluid. From the central nervous system and outward, the three membranes are the pia mater, the arachnoid mater, and the dura mater. When the term **leptomeninges** is used, it refers to the pia and arachnoid mater together.

Pia mater

This is the innermost layer of the meninges and it adheres tightly to the surfaces of the underlying structures, covering all the gyri and even dips into all the sulci. Its name reflects this careful hugging; it is Latin for gentle or tender mother.

Arachnoid mater

The arachnoid mater (so named because of the similarity of its structure to a spider's web) lies above and roughly follows the outline of the pia mater, although it doesn't dip down into the sulci.

The space between the pia and arachnoid mater is called the subarachnoidal space. It is filled with cerebrospinal fluid.

Dura mater

The dura mater is the toughest of the meningeal membranes (it is therefore called, in Latin, the tough mother). In the cranium, it has two layers, the outer **periosteal** and the inner **meningeal**; in the spinal cord, it only has one layer.

In addition to housing the blood-carrying **sinus** structures (see the next chapter), it dips into the brain to separate certain structures from each other.

These separations are the **falx cerebri** (separating the two cerebral hemispheres), the **falx cerebelli** (separating the two cerebellar hemispheres posteriorly), the **tentorium cerebelli** (separating the cerebellum from the occipital lobes of the cerebrum), and the **diaphragma sellae**, a roof-like structure covering the pituitary gland in the hypophyseal fossa of the sella turcica; it has a small superior opening where the pituitary stalk passes.

The potential spaces below and above the dura mater are known as the **subdural** and **epidural** spaces, respectively. Injuries to the **bridging veins** found in the subdural space may give rise to a **subdural hematoma** (bleeding). An **epidural hematoma**, on the other hand, is typically a result of trauma to the temporal region of the head, causing the **middle meningeal artery** to rupture.

Chapter 3

Arteries and Veins

Arteries

The two pairs of arteries that supply the brain with oxygenated blood are the **internal carotid arteries** and the **vertebral arteries**. They are branches of branches from the aorta, and are sometimes referred to as the **anterior** and **posterior circulation**, respectively.

Internal carotid arteries

The **right internal carotid artery** is a branch of the **right common carotid artery**, which is a branch of the **brachiocephalic trunk**, which is a branch of the **arch of the aorta**.

The **left internal carotid artery** is a branch of the **left common carotid artery**, which is a branch of the **arch of the aorta**.

The internal carotid arteries enter the cranium through the **carotid canal**.

The two major branches of the internal carotid arteries are the **anterior** and **middle cerebral arteries**.

Vertebral arteries

The right and left vertebral arteries are branches of the right and left **subclavian arteries**, respectively (subclavian = below the clavicle).

The **right** subclavian artery, like the right common carotid artery, is a branch of the **brachiocephalic trunk**.

The **left** subclavian artery, like the left common carotid artery, is a branch of the **arch of the aorta** (left/distal to the left common carotid artery).

Once they have branched off from the subclavian arteries, they run in the **transversal foramina** of the upper six cervical vertebrae. They enter the cranium via **foramen magnum**.

The vertebral arteries join each other roughly where the medulla oblongata meets the pons, and give rise to the **basilar artery**, which runs in the midline of the anterior side of the pons.

When the basilar artery reaches the point where the pons meets the mesencephalon, it branches into the **posterior cerebral arteries** and also gives rise to several branches before that (see below).

The circle of Willis

Through thin communicating arteries, the branches of the internal carotid arteries and the vertebral arteries form a structure known as the circle of Willis. The circle that is created is found at the base of the brain, and it encircles (in rostral to caudal order) the optic chiasm, the pituitary gland, and the mammillary bodies.

The **posterior communicating arteries** run between the **posterior cerebral arteries** and the **internal carotid arteries** (before these branch into the anterior and middle cerebral arteries); they are the connections between the anterior and posterior circulations.

The **anterior communicating artery** runs between the **anterior cerebral arteries**, and thus connects the left and right sides of the anterior circulation.

So, the complete circle is formed by the **left anterior cerebral artery**, the **left internal carotid artery**, the **left posterior communicating artery**, the **left posterior cerebral artery** that connects to the **right posterior cerebral artery** via the bifurcation of the basilar artery, and from there the circle continues with the **right posterior communicating artery**, the **right internal carotid artery**, the **right anterior cerebral artery**, which connects to our starting point via the **anterior communicating artery**.

The cerebral arteries

The areas covered by the **three pairs** of cerebral arteries are roughly as follows:

The **anterior cerebral artery** supplies the **medial** parts of the **frontal** and **parietal** lobes, including a small strip **su-**

periorly, to the left and right of the longitudinal fissure.

The **middle cerebral artery** supplies the **lateral** parts of the **frontal** and **parietal** lobes, as well as the **superior** parts of the **temporal** lobes.

The **posterior cerebral artery** supplies the **occipital** lobes and the **inferior** parts of the **temporal** lobes.

Important branches to the cerebellum

There are **three major branches** from the vertebral and basilar arteries to the **cerebellum**.

The **first** branch arises from the vertebral arteries in the level of the medulla oblongata, before the vertebral arteries join and become the basilar artery. This branch is called the **posterior inferior cerebellar artery** (PICA).

The **second** branch arises from the basilar artery shortly after it has been "created." This branch is called the **anterior inferior cerebellar artery** (AICA).

The **third** branch arises from the basilar artery just before it branches into the posterior cerebral arteries. This branch is called the **superior cerebellar artery**.

So there are three important branches to the cerebellum - one superior and two (anterior and posterior) inferior. All of these branches come from the posterior circulation.

Branches to the brain stem

The brain stem receives its blood from branches of the vertebral and basilar arteries, as well as from branches of the cerebellar arteries.

Blood supply of the spinal cord

Two arterial branches leave from the medial aspects of the vertebral arteries and join in the midline of the anterior medulla oblongata to become the **anterior spinal artery**, that then descends caudally to supply the anterior part (the anterior two-thirds) of the spinal cord.

Two **posterior spinal arteries** leave from either the vertebral arteries or from the posterior inferior cerebellar arteries (PICA); they continue caudally as separate branches (or rather as a network) and do not join and become one artery in the midline.

Both the anterior and the posterior spinal arteries are continually being "reinforced" or "refilled" by other branches throughout their way to the most caudal parts of the spinal cord.

The artery of Adamkiewicz is a particularly large branch that reinforces the anterior spinal artery; it is most often seen on the left side, at the level of the lowest thoracic vertebrae.

Veins and sinuses

Veins and sinuses carry venous blood from the brain out of the cranium and back to the heart and lungs. The veins are basically similar to veins in other parts of the body (although here they lack valves), but the sinuses are unique to the intracranial vascular arrangement - they are blood-transporting structures formed between the layers of the dura mater. They do, however, communicate with the veins, and together they build an elaborately interconnected system of vessels. This system is complicated, but some of its central components will be discussed.

One way of approaching this topic is to start at the end and work our way backwards.

The venous blood leaves the cranium through the left and right **internal jugular veins** (which pass through the jugular foramen). How does it reach these veins?

The blood reaches the internal jugular veins mainly through the **sigmoid sinus** on both sides. The sigmoid sinus is a roughly S-shaped structure that is found approximately posterolateral to the jugular foramen.

The blood reaches the sigmoid sinus through the **transverse sinus**. This is an almost straight structure that runs from the posterior midpoint of the cranium towards the sigmoid sinus.

The blood reaches the transverse sinus from the **confluence of sinuses**, found near the internal occipital protuberance.

The confluence of sinuses is a structure that collects blood from several other sinuses:

1: **Superior sagittal sinus** (which follows the cranial attachment of the falx cerebri and thus runs in the superior midline of the cranial cavity).

2: **Straight sinus** (which receives blood from the **inferior sagittal sinus,** which runs in the lower/deeper part of the falx cerebri, and also from the **great cerebral vein**, also known as the **vein of Galen**).

3: **Occipital sinus**, which runs from approximately the foramen magnum and in the inferior posterior midline of the cranium.

So, three sinus structures join at the confluence of sinuses at the back of the cranium, and from there, blood flows to the left and right transverse and sigmoid sinuses and out from the cranium via the internal jugular veins.

It appears to be the case that the superior sagittal sinus most often empties into the right transverse sinus, and the straight sinus most often empties into the left transverse sinus (in other words, there isn't always a mixing of their blood in the confluence of sinuses).

On the lateral sides of the sella turcica are the **cavernous sinuses**, two important structures containing not just venous blood (from the **ophthalmic veins, superficial middle cerebral veins** and the **sphenoparietal sinuses**) but also cranial nerves (**III**, **IV**, first and second branch of **V**, and **VI**) as well as a portion of the **internal carotid artery**.

From these cavernous sinuses, blood flows to the internal jugular vein via the **inferior petrosal sinus**, and to the sigmoid or transverse sinus via the **superior petrosal sinus**. There is also communication with the **basilar plexus**, a network of veins that lies more or less on the clivus.

The veins of the cerebrum are divided into groups of **superficial** and **deep cerebral veins**.

In the superficial (also called "external") group, you find:

1: The **superior cerebral veins** that drain mostly into the superior sagittal sinus.

2: The **superficial middle cerebral veins** that drain mostly into the cavernous sinus.

3: The **inferior cerebral veins** that drain mostly into the transverse sinus.

In the deep group, you find:

1: The left and right **internal cerebral veins** that unite with the **basal vein** (also known as the **vein of Rosenthal**) and become the **great cerebral vein** (also known as the **vein of Galen**).

2: The great cerebral vein then flows into the **straight sinus** (together with the inferior sagittal sinus) which flows into the confluence of sinuses.

If you get an opportunity to study these complex networks with models or 3D images - take it. It is almost impossible to understand through text and 2D images only.

Arachnoid granulations

There are protrusions from the subarachnoid space that bulge into the sinuses on many places, most notably into the superior sagittal sinus. These protrusions are called **arachnoid granulations** and through them, cerebrospinal fluid can be drained from the subarachnoid space into the blood circulation.

Chapter 4

The Ventricular System and CSF

The ventricular system and the subarachnoid space in the rest of the central nervous system is filled with **cerebrospinal fluid** (CSF).

This is a fluid with several functions, such as allowing the brain to float around inside the cranium instead of being pressed against the cranial walls by the force of gravity.

CSF is produced by a structure called **choroid plexus**, that is found in the walls of the ventricles. It is drained into the blood circulation mainly through the **arachnoid granulations** (see the previous chapter).

The ventricular system

The ventricular system consists of the **four ventricles** (**two lateral** ventricles, and then the **third** and the **fourth** ventricles) including the **central canal** of the spinal cord, and their various connections, and it communicates with the subarachnoid space and associated cisterns mainly via **three apertures**.

The **two lateral ventricles** lie in the left and right cerebral hemispheres. They have a body and three "**horns**" - **anterior, posterior**, and **inferior** - and these horns give the ventricles their shape (which, if viewed from the right side, is something like the letter C, with a little "tail" in the middle of its left side).

The anterior horns stretch into the **frontal lobes**, the posterior horns stretch into the **occipital lobes**, and the inferior horns stretch into the **temporal lobes**.

The lateral ventricles do not communicate directly with each other (the anterior horns lie close but are separated by a thin wall known as the **septum pellucidum**), but they both connect to the third ventricle via the **left** and **right interventricular foramina** (**foramina of Monro**). These foramina extend from the **anterior horns** of the lateral ventricles.

The **third ventricle** lies in the midline, roughly between the left and right thalamus. Many but not all people have an **interthalamic adhesion** that extends between the left and right thalamus through the third ventricle. In addition to the two interventricular foramina, it has a connection to the fourth ventricle via the **cerebral aqueduct** (**the aqueduct of Sylvius**).

The **fourth ventricle** lies between the cerebellum and pons/medulla oblongata. It is continuous with the central canal of the spinal cord (the point in the medulla oblongata at which this transition takes place is called the **obex**), and also has **three apertures** that connect the ventricular system to the subarachnoid space and cisterns: The **two lat-**

eral apertures (foramina of **Luschka**) extending out from both sides, and the **median aperture** (foramen of **Magendie**), found roughly in the lower posterior midline of the fourth ventricle.

Development

During the embryological period, the precursor to the central nervous system consists of a neural tube, and the hollow center of the tube becomes the ventricular system.

In caudal to rostral order:

The **caudal part** becomes the **central canal** of the spinal cord.

The **rhombencephalon** (precursor to cerebellum, pons and medulla oblongata) gives rise to the **fourth ventricle**.

The **mesencephalon** gives rise to the **cerebral aqueduct**.

The **diencephalon** gives rise to the **third ventricle**.

The **telencephalon** gives rise to the **lateral ventricles**.

Chapter 5

Spinal Cord

The spinal cord is a continuation of the medulla oblongata that stretches caudally all the way down to approximately the first two lumbar vertebrae (L1-L2).

It is surrounded and protected by the vertebral column, which of course continues further with the rest of the lumbar, as well as the sacral and coccygeal, vertebrae.

While the spinal cord itself ends at L1-L2, it gives off nerves that "hang down" within the most caudal parts of the vertebral column, and these nerves give rise to lower lumbar, sacral and coccygeal nerves. Due to its resemblance to the tail of a horse, this bundle of nerves is called the **cauda equina**.

The most caudal part of the spinal cord is tapered and is known as the **conus medullaris**.

There is also a thin structure formed by connective tissue

that hangs down from the conus medullaris, known as the **filum terminale**.

Similar to the rest of the central nervous system, the spinal cord is surrounded by the three layers of meninges (pia, arachnoid and dura mater).

In the posterior midline of the spinal cord there is a **posterior median sulcus**, and in the anterior midline there is an **anterior median fissure**; the fissure is wider than the sulcus.

The spinal cord, just like the cerebrum, has both **white** and **grey matter**.

In an axial (transverse) section, the grey matter is found in the center as a symmetric structure that is often compared to a butterfly or the letter H. Its shape varies slightly throughout the length of the spinal cord, but the general form is retained.

The white matter is peripheral to and surrounds the grey matter.

The grey matter contains the cell bodies of neurons, while the white matter mostly consists of the long axons of neurons.

The grey matter

In the middle of the H, and thus in the middle of the spinal cord, is the **central canal**. It contains cerebrospinal fluid and is continuous with the fourth ventricle and the rest of the ventricular system.

The thinner middle part of the H that connects the left and

right sides (and that surrounds the central canal) is known as the **grey commissure**.

The H has two "points" pointing backwards and two "points" pointing forwards. These are known as the **dorsal** and **ventral horns**, respectively (the terms posterior and anterior horns are sometimes used, and sometimes the term "column" is used instead of "horn").

In addition to dorsal and ventral horns, some parts of the grey matter (usually the thoracic and the most rostral/cranial parts of the lumbar spinal cord) have **lateral horns** as well, bulging out to the sides, lateral to the central canal.

The **dorsal horns** receive **afferent** signals coming in to the spinal cord through the **dorsal roots**.

The **ventral horns** give rise to **efferent** signals exiting the spinal cord through the **ventral roots**.

The dorsal root has a swelling that is called the **dorsal ganglion**, that contains cell bodies of neurons.

The dorsal and ventral roots are joined together to create the **spinal nerves**.

Thus, even though these signals are separated in the spinal cord, the spinal nerves contain both afferent and efferent nerves.

There are **31 pairs of spinal nerves** (8 cervical, 12 thoracic, 5 lumbar, 5 sacral, and 1 coccygeal).

The white matter

In the white matter, neurons are arranged in various tracts, running in rostral/cranial (ascending) and caudal (descending) direction.

There are many tracts in the spinal cord, and each contains a bundle of nerves carrying specific information that is to be delivered to a specific location.

Their directions are usually reflected in their names - for example, a corticospinal tract runs from the cortex to the spine, and a spinocerebellar tract runs from the spine to the cerebellum.

The largest **descending tracts** are:

The **lateral corticospinal tracts**. These lie in the posterolateral spinal cord, between the grey matter and the posterior spinocerebellar tract.

The **anterior corticospinal tracts**. These lie in the anteromedial spinal cord, to the left and right of the anterior median fissure.

The lateral and anterior corticospinal tracts are known as the **pyramidal tracts**. The **extrapyramidal tracts** include the rubrospinal, olivospinal, vestibulospinal and reticulospinal tracts (be aware, though, that these tracts may have different names depending on which source you use).

The largest **ascending tracts** are:

The **dorsal/posterior columns**, consisting of the left and right **fasciculus gracilis** and the **fasciculus cuneatus**. These lie in the posteromedial compartment, with the fasciculus gracilis being the most medial. A rule of thumb is that the fasciculus gracilis carries information from the lower half of the body and the fasciculus cuneatus carries information from the upper half. When they reach the level of the medulla oblongata, they become the **medial lemniscal system**.

The **lateral** and **anterior spinothalamic tracts**. These lie medial to the anterior spinocerebellar tracts and lateral to the anterior corticospinal tracts, respectively. When they reach the brainstem, they are known as the **spinal lemniscus**.

The **posterior** and **anterior spinocerebellar tracts** - these lie in the postero- and anterolateral rims of the white matter, respectively.

Decussation

Most tracts, whether they are ascending or descending, cross over ("**decussate**") to the other side (left to right, right to left).

This is why the **left cerebral hemisphere** processes both motor signals to and sensory signals from the **right side of the body**.

This decussation is to a large extent done in the **medulla oblongata**.

However, there are exceptions. One important exception is the **lateral** and **anterior spinothalamic tracts**. The neurons in these tracts (that carry information about pain and temperature, and some touch and pressure, respectively) **cross over already when they enter the spinal cord** (often they ascend a few levels, in the tract of Lissauer, before they decussate, however).

The sensory information that is transported via the dorsal columns (fine touch, vibration and proprioception) switches sides in the medulla oblongata, which gives rise to the peculiar situation that damage to one side of the spinal cord may cause symptoms from both the left and right sides of the body.

This is known as the **Brown-Séquard syndrome**. Suppose that the entire left half of the spinal cord is injured at a lower thoracic level. Which tracts from which sides are involved?

The majority of the motor signals (lateral corticospinal tract) crosses over at the medulla oblongata; damage to the left side of the spinal cord thus causes loss of motor signals to and paralysis of the left leg.

The sensory signals carried in the dorsal columns also cross over at the level of the medulla oblongata; damage to the left side of the spinal cord thus causes loss of fine touch, vibration and proprioception from the left leg.

The sensory signals carried in the spinothalamic tracts, however, cross over at about the level of the spinal cord where they enter; damage to the left side of the spinal cord thus causes loss of pain and temperature from the right leg.

The **anterior corticospinal tracts** also decussate at the level of the spinal cord, not in the medulla oblongata.

Another exception is the **cerebellum**, where the left side processes signals from the left side of the body (no decussation).

Chapter 6

Brainstem

Mesencephalon

When viewed dorsally, two pairs of bulges are apparent on the mesencephalic surface. These are divided into one superior pair and one inferior pair, called the **superior colliculi** and the **inferior colliculi**, respectively. Together, they are known as the **corpora quadrigemina**.

(The **pineal gland** is also visible in this view, hanging superior to the superior colliculi, in the midline.)

The colliculi are part of the **tectum**, the **dorsal** part of the mesencephalon. The **ventral** part (ventral to the aqueduct of Sylvius) is dominated by the **cerebral peduncles**.

The ventral part of the cerebral peduncles consists of the **crura cerebri** (one crus, many crura), and dorsal to them is the **tegmentum**. Descending motor signals from the cerebral cortex pass through the crura cerebri on their way to the spinal cord (the corticospinal tract).

Between the crura cerebri and the tegmentum is the **substantia nigra**, which produces **dopamine** and is a part of the **basal ganglia**.

Dorsal and medial to the substantia nigra, in the superior tegmental area, is the **red nucleus**.

The nuclei to CN III and CN IV (**oculomotor** and **trochlear** nerves, respectively) lie in the medial parts, ventral to the aqueduct. CN III is found roughly in the level of the superior colliculi, and CN IV is found roughly in the level of the inferior colliculi.

Pons

The **dorsal** part of the pons is called the **tegmentum** (note that the tegmentum in the mesencephalon is ventral; however, the pontine and mesencephalic tegmenti are still continuous).

One important structure in the dorsal pons is the **locus coeruleus** (several alternate spellings exist). It is found in the rostral and dorsal part of pons, close to the wall of the fourth ventricle. Here, **norepinephrine**-producing neurons are found.

The **ventral** part of the pons is called the **base**. In the superficial ventral midline is the **basilar sulcus** where the **basilar artery** runs.

The **cerebellopontine angle** is a lateral space that arises where the pons, the cerebellum, and the medulla oblongata meet. Here, CN VII and CN VIII (the facial and vestibulocochlear nerves, respectively) exit.

In addition to CN VII and CN VIII, CN VI (the abducens nerve) also exits the brainstem in the junction between the pons and the medulla oblongata. CN VI exits medially while the other two exit laterally.

The fourth cranial nerve to exit from the pons is the large trigeminal nerve (CN V). It exits roughly in the mid-level, on the lateral side.

Medulla oblongata

The medulla oblongata is continuous with the spinal cord, and the **posterior median sulcus** and **anterior median fissure** of the spinal cord continue in the medulla oblongata.

On the lateral sides of the anterior median fissure are two swellings called the **pyramids**.

Lateral to the pyramids are the **ventrolateral sulci**, and lateral to these sulci are the **olives**, which also are bilateral swellings of the medulla oblongata.

The olives are separated from the **inferior cerebellar peduncles** by the **dorsolateral sulci**.

The ventrolateral sulcus is also known as the anterolateral sulcus or pre-olivary sulcus.

The dorsolateral sulcus is also known as the posterolateral sulcus or the post- or retro-olivary sulcus.

The hypoglossal nerve (cranial nerve XII) exits the medulla oblongata via the ventrolateral sulcus, and the glossopharyngeal, vagus and accessory nerves (cranial nerves IX, X and XI, respectively) exit via the dorsolateral sulcus.

The pyramids are formed by the **pyramidal/corticospinal tracts**, and the olives are formed by the **inferior olivary nuclei**.

The **decussations** of the pyramids are located in the caudal parts of the medulla oblongata.

Three important tracts and their way through the brainstem

Corticospinal tract (descending)

Cerebrum: The signals originate in the **motor areas** in the **frontal lobe,** and travel through the **corona radiata** and continue in the **internal capsule**.

Mesencephalon: They continue in the ipsilateral **crus cerebri** in the **cerebral peduncle**.

Pons: The signals travel via the medial and slightly anterior parts of the pons.

Medulla oblongata: The signals travel in the **pyramid**, where they also **decussate** and continue on the contralateral side.

Spinal cord: The signals travel in (mainly) the **lateral corticospinal tract**.

Spinothalamic tract (ascending)

Spinal cord: The signals (in this example, pain signals) come in from the periphery, enter the spinal cord via the dorsal root and horn, and **almost immediately decussate**. They then ascend via the contralateral **lateral spinothalamic tract**.

Medulla oblongata, pons and mesencephalon: In the brainstem, these signals travel in what is known as the **spinal lemniscus**.

Cerebrum: The signals reach the **thalamus**, and from there continue to the **somatosensory cortex (parietal lobe)**.

Dorsal columns/medial lemniscus (ascending)

Spinal cord: The signals (in this example, proprioception signals) come in from the periphery, enter the spinal cord via the dorsal root and horn, and ascend in the ipsilateral **dorsal columns** (signals from the lower limb in the medial **fasciculus gracilis**, and signals from the upper limb in the more lateral **fasciculus cuneatus**).

Medulla oblongata: The signals reach the **nucleus gracilis** (or **nucleus cuneatus**), **decussate**, and continue in the brainstem tract known as the **medial lemniscus**.

Pons and mesencephalon: The tract is known as the **medial lemniscus** in these brainstem parts as well.

Cerebrum: The signals reach the **thalamus**, and from there continue to the **somatosensory cortex (parietal lobe)**.

Chapter 7

Cranial Nerves

There are 12 pairs of cranial nerves, most of which have their nuclei in the brain stem. They are usually referred to as CN followed by a roman numeral (I-XII). We will go through them one by one and then finish off with an assortment of additional facts. (Some cranial nerves have many functions, and not all of them will be listed; also, their nuclei are not always as clearly demarcated as this text might indicate.)

CN I: Olfactory nerve

This nerve, seen as two long projections with terminal bulbs on the anterior inferior side of the brain, is sending signals to the central nervous system from olfactory (smell) receptors in the nasal cavity. The olfactory nerve doesn't have a nucleus in the brain stem, but instead sends its signals directly to several places such as the **piriform cortex**, the **orbitofrontal cortex**, and the **limbic system**.

CN II: Optic nerve

This nerve is sending visual signals from the **retina** of the eyes to the **occipital cortex**.

From the retina, the nerve passes through the **optic canal**, then reaches the X-shaped **optic chiasma** where some of its fibers cross over while other fibers will continue on the same side. After the chiasma, the nerves continue as the **optic tracts**.

Signals from the medial/nasal retina cross over in the chiasma, and signals from the lateral/temporal retina continue on the same side.

In other words, signals from objects in the right side of the right eye's field of vision will "land" on the right medial/nasal retina, and they will cross over to the left optic tract. Signals from the left side will "land" on the right lateral/temporal retina, and will continue ipsilaterally.

Due to this partial crossover, the right optic tract will carry information about the left field of vision (it has uncrossed information from the right lateral/temporal retina and crossed information from the left medial/nasal retina). Obviously, the left optic tract will carry information about the right field of vision.

The optic tracts synapse in the **thalamus**, and from there continue in the so-called **optic radiation** that terminates in the **occipital cortex**.

There are additional routes for visual signals. One of these is responsible for the pupillary light reflex. After leaving the optic chiasma, some signals reach the Edinger-Westphal nucleus in the mesencephalon instead of going to the thalamus. From there, efferent signals are sent out so that both the left and right pupils constrict (even if the signal has come from only one of the eyes).

CN III: Oculomotor nerve

This nerve controls **four of the six extraocular muscles** (superior/inferior/medial rectus muscles plus the inferior oblique muscle).

It has a **nucleus in the mesencephalon**, and it sends out fibers that reach the orbit and the extraocular muscles via the **cavernous sinus** and the **superior orbital fissure**.

It also controls the **levator palpebrae superioris** muscle (which lifts the eyelid), and has **parasympathetic fibers** that emerge from the **Edinger-Westphal nucleus** that are involved in pupillary constriction and accommodation.

CN IV: Trochlear nerve

This nerve has a **nucleus in the mesencephalon** and passes, just like the oculomotor nerve, the **cavernous sinus** and the **superior orbital fissure** on its way to the orbit.

It controls the **superior oblique muscle**, one of the six extraocular muscles.

CN V: Trigeminal nerve

This is the largest of the cranial nerves, and its system of nuclei stretches through the whole brainstem and the upper parts of the spinal cord; its exit point from the brainstem, however, is from the mid-pons.

Before splitting up into its divisions and leaving the cranium, it gives rise to a ganglion (trigeminal/semilunar/gasserian ganglion) in the middle cranial fossa.

It has three major divisions: **Ophthalmic**, **maxillary** and **mandibular** (usually referred to as **V1**, **V2** and **V3**, respectively).

It mainly handles sensory information from the scalp and from the face, including some interior structures. They cover the following areas, roughly:

V1, ophthalmic: Superior scalp, forehead, upper eyelids, medial nose.
Leaves cranium through **superior orbital fissure**.

V2, maxillary: Lower eyelid, lateral nose, upper teeth and lip, anterior cheek and anterior temporal region.
Leaves cranium through **foramen rotundum**.

V3, mandibular: Lower teeth and lip, chin, posterior cheek, temporal scalp. This branch also innervates the muscles of mastication.
Leaves cranium through **foramen ovale**.

CN VI: Abducens nerve

This nerve has a **nucleus in the pons** and passes, just like the oculomotor and trochlear nerves, the **cavernous sinus** and the **superior orbital fissure** on its way to the orbit.

It controls the **lateral rectus muscle**, one of the six extraocular muscles. Like the nerve's name implies, this muscle abducts the eye (pulls it laterally).

CN VII: Facial nerve

This nerve innervates the muscles of the face and also handles taste signals from the anterior two-thirds of the tongue.

It has a **nucleus in the pons**, begins to exit the cranium through the **internal acoustic meatus** from where it continues to run inside bones before it exits through the **stylomastoid foramen**.

From there it enters the parotid gland, and it then splits up into five major branches: **Temporal**, **zygomatic**, **buccal**, **mandibular** and **cervical**.

The branch of the facial nerve that transmits taste signals from the anterior two-thirds of the tongue is called **chorda tympani**.

CN VIII: Vestibulocochlear nerve

This nerve consists of two parts, the **vestibular** and the **cochlear nerve**. Most sources are rather unclear about the exact location of the nuclei of these nerves, but most place them around the border between the **pons** and the **medulla oblongata**.

They both exit the cranium through the **internal acoustic meatus** and continue to the inner ear.

The vestibular nerve transmits information about equilibrium/balance, and the cochlear nerve transmits auditory signals.

CN IX: Glossopharyngeal nerve

This nerve has its **nucleus in the medulla oblongata**, leaves the cranium through the **jugular foramen**, and has both motor and sensory parts.

It is notably responsible for sensation in the pharynx (including the uvula and taste from the posterior one-third of the tongue) and for innervating the stylopharyngeus muscle that assists in swallowing.

CN X: Vagus nerve

This cranial nerve is unique in that it not only innervates structures in the head and neck, but also connects to organs in the thoracic and abdominal cavities. It constitutes a large portion of the parasympathetic nervous system.

The vagus nerve is associated with a group of nuclei in the **medulla oblongata**, such as the **dorsal motor nucleus of the vagus**, the **nucleus ambiguus**, and the **solitary nucleus**.

It exits the cranium through the **jugular foramen**, and shortly thereafter forms two ganglia - the **superior**, or **jugular**, **ganglion**, and the **inferior**, or **nodose**, **ganglion**.

One of many relevant branches is the **recurrent laryngeal nerves**, so named because while the vagus nerve descends from the neck into the thoracic cavity, these branches then make a turn and ascend back into the neck again. On the **right** side, the nerve makes a turn around the **right subclavian artery** before it ascends again, and on the **left** side it makes a turn around the **arch of the aorta**. The recurrent laryngeal nerves innervate many structures of the **larynx**.

CN XI: Accessory nerve

This nerve has two roots, one **spinal root** and one **cranial root**.

The spinal root comes from the upper parts of the cervical spinal cord, and ascends **into the cranium** through the **foramen magnum**, where it joins the cranial root.

The cranial root originates from the **medulla oblongata**, and exits the medulla oblongata through the retro-olivary sulcus.

Together, these nerves exit the cranium through the **jugular foramen**, and innervate the **sternocleidomastoid** and **trapezius** muscles.

Note that this is the way it has usually been taught - there appears to be some controversy that is yet unsolved, and while no textbook that I have consulted has switched to the new viewpoint entirely, it is good to keep in mind and be open to changes.

CN XII: Hypoglossal nerve

This nerve has its **nucleus in the medulla oblongata**. It exits the medulla oblongata in the **sulcus between the pyramid and the olive**, and exits the cranium through the **hypoglossal canal**.

It is responsible for the movements of the tongue.

Some general facts

In chapters about the cranial nerves in textbooks, the brain is often viewed from an anteroinferior perspective, so that all the nerves' exit points from the brain stem are visualized. At first glance, it is something like a chaos, but if one groups them together, they will be easier to remember.

For example, let's start by looking at the four most inferior cranial nerves (CN IX-XII). They all exit the brain stem from the medulla. Remember that there is a ventrolateral and a dorsolateral sulcus between the pyramid and the olive, and the olive and the inferior cerebellar peduncle, respectively.

CN XII exits in the ventrolateral sulcus.
CN IX, **X** and **XI** (cranial part) exit in the dorsolateral sulcus.

We continue with the next three nerves - VI, VII, and VIII. They exit the brainstem roughly between the pons and the medulla oblongata.

CN VI exits medially, close to the midline.
CN VII and **VIII** exit laterally (VIII most laterally).

So - we're already done with seven of the twelve nerves and it turned out to be very easy. And the first two cranial nerves do not have brainstem nuclei, so you only have three more to learn; this is perfectly achievable.

CN V exits laterally at the mid-pons level; it is a big one and almost impossible to miss.

CN IV actually exits from the posterior side of the midbrain (and is the only cranial nerve that truly decussates, according to most sources). It makes a turn and comes over to the anterior side, superior to CN V.

CN III exits medially from the midbrain and runs between the posterior cerebral artery and the superior cerebellar artery.

CN I and **II** should be easy to identify on these images.

Medial longitudinal fasciculus

This is a brainstem structure, often referred to as MLF, that synchronizes the actions of cranial nerves **III**, **IV** and **VI**, so that eye movements may be smooth and so that the gaze can remain fixed on a particular object even though the head is shifting its position.

Brainstem reflexes

The pupillary light reflex is mentioned above. It is one of three important brainstem reflexes that together allow you to assess large parts of the brainstem even if the patient is unconscious; if these reflexes work, then much of the brainstem is actually still alive, which is very valuable information in a coma situation. The afferent (A) and efferent (E) parts of the reflexes are listed.

Pupillary light reflex:
A: CN II (optic nerve)
E: CN III (oculomotor nerve)

Corneal reflex:
A: CN V (trigeminal nerve)
E: CN VII (facial nerve)

Gag reflex:
A: CN IX (glossopharyngeal nerve)
E: CN X (vagus nerve)

Mnemonics

There are many mnemonics to help students remember the names and order of the cranial nerves. The one that I was taught during medical school is the following slightly naughty sentence:

Oh, oh, oh - to touch and feel virgin girls' vagina - AH!
(Another version replaced "AH" with "and hymen.")

Another mnemonic was taught in order to remember which cranial nerves were primarily **s**ensory, primarily **mo**tor, or **b**oth:

Some say money matters, but my brother says big boobs matter more.
(Another version replaced "boobs" with "brains.")

Chapter 8

Cerebellum

The cerebellum ("little brain") is situated in the **posterior cranial fossa**, and is separated from the occipital lobes of the cerebrum by the **tentorium cerebelli**.

It is attached to the brainstem in front of it via three **peduncles**, that allow afferent and efferent signals to travel between the cerebellum and the rest of the nervous system:

Superior cerebellar peduncles connect it to the **mesencephalon**.
Middle cerebellar peduncles connect it to the **pons**.
Inferior cerebellar peduncles connect it to the **medulla oblongata**.

Similar to the cerebrum, the cerebellum has **two hemispheres** (left and right). In the midline, the hemispheres are connected by a structure called the **vermis** (which, however, the cerebrum does not have).

And like the cerebrum it has a cortex made up of grey matter, below which is the white matter, that houses deep nuclei.

On the surface it has roughly horizontally running gyri-like thin and small ridges called **folia** (one folium, many folia).

Parallel with the folia are slightly deeper fissures that divide the cerebellum into **lobules**, that are grouped together into **three lobes**.

When discussing this, the cerebellum is usually "unfolded" so that it is pictured as a butterfly, with the vermis as the body and the hemispheres as the wings; the anterior part is then at the top of the drawing, and the posterior part at the bottom.

The three most anterior lobules form the **anterior lobe**.
The next five lobules form the **posterior lobe**.
The most posterior lobule is the **nodule**, which has two lateral attachments (left and right **flocculus**, together the **flocculi**), and together they form the **flocculonodular lobe**.

Separating the anterior lobe from the posterior lobe is the **primary fissure**.

Separating the posterior lobe from the flocculonodular lobe is the **posterolateral fissure**.

In the posterior lobe, there is also a rather large **horizontal fissure**. However, this fissure does not seem to divide the cerebellum in a clinically or physiologically significant way.

Note that the hemispheres **and** the vermis are included in the lobes.

Sometimes, the cerebellum is divided into sections in a different way (vertical instead of horizontal), using the terms vestibulocerebellum, spinocerebellum and cerebrocerebellum.

Vestibulocerebellum is the flocculonodular lobe.
Spinocerebellum is the vermis and the most medial parts of the hemispheres.
Cerebrocerebellum is the lateral parts of the hemispheres.

Deep in the white matter of the hemispheres are four deep nuclei. From lateral to medial, they are:

Dentate nucleus.
Emboliform nucleus.
Globose nucleus.
Fastigial nucleus.

The emboliform and globose nuclei are sometimes grouped together and called the **interposed nucleus**.

Normally, only the dentate nucleus is visible in sections or on imaging.

The medial and inferior parts of the posterior lobe contain two bulging structures that are close to the foramen magnum. They are known as the **cerebellar tonsils**.

Arbor vitae is a term that often shows up in descriptions of the cerebellum. It is Latin for "tree of life," and refers to the branching pattern produced by the white matter on some sections.

Chapter 9

Cerebral Hemispheres (Surface)

There are parts of the cerebrum that are clearly seen on the surface, and other parts that are only visible after sectioning (or through imaging). We start by mapping out the surface, and then in the next chapter go deeper, looking at the anatomy with sagittal and coronal sections.

Structures seen on the surface

The cerebral hemispheres are divided into **four pairs of lobes - frontal**, **parietal**, **temporal** and **occipital**. The lobes are demarcated by fissures or sulci.

The most conspicuous fissure, however, is the **longitudinal fissure** that separates the left and right hemispheres. It runs all the way from the anterior to the posterior aspects of the cerebrum.

The **central sulcus** (sometimes called the Rolandic fissure) separates the frontal lobe from the parietal lobe.

The **lateral sulcus** (sometimes called the Sylvian fissure) separates the temporal lobe from the frontal and parietal lobes.

The **parietooccipital sulcus** separates the parietal lobe from the occipital lobe. Within the occipital lobe, on its medial side and roughly perpendicular to the parietooccipital sulcus, is another sulcus called the **calcarine sulcus**.

Aside from these structures, there are many gyri on the surface of the brain.

Some conspicuous gyri

At first glance, the gyri on the surface of the brain seem to be arranged like a completely random landscape, but there is actually some consistency to it, and when you compare different brains, you will find that although they are different, some patterns recur. Now, these patterns are not always apparent in every case, but they exist, at least in theory - and the theory is a little something like this:

Gyri of the frontal lobe

Immediately in front of the central sulcus is the **precentral gyrus**. It runs more or less parallel to the central sulcus. In front if it is the **precentral sulcus**.

In front of the precentral gyrus, and more or less perpendicular to it, are **three frontal gyri**. All of them have logical names - one is superior to the others (superior and medial, next to the longitudinal fissure), another is inferior to the others, and the third is obviously in the middle. Naturally, these gyri are called the **superior**, the **middle** and the **inferior frontal gyrus**.

Note that the middle frontal gyrus is not the same as the **medial frontal gyrus**, which is found on the medial side of the frontal lobe. It is found between the lobe's superior aspect and the **cingulate sulcus** and the **cingulate gyrus** (which is riding on top of the corpus callosum). (In some sources, what here is called the medial frontal gyrus is included in the term superior frontal gyrus, however.)

Looking from the inferior side of the brain, identifying the **straight gyrus** is easy. It runs immediately next to, and parallel to, the longitudinal fissure and the olfactory nerves.

Lateral to the straight gyrus is a group of **four orbital gyri**. The orbital sulci that mark the borders of these gyri lie in a pattern that is often compared to the letter H. Based on this, the orbital gyri are then given logical names.

Medial to the H is the **medial orbital gyrus**.
Lateral to the H is the **lateral orbital gyrus**.
Anterior to the middle bar of the H is the **anterior orbital gyrus**.
Posterior to the middle bar of the H is the **posterior orbital gyrus**.

Gyri of the temporal lobe

There are three more or less horizontally running gyri on the lateral side of the temporal lobe, and they all have logical names:

The most superior gyrus (immediately below the lateral sulcus) is the **superior temporal gyrus**.
Below it is the **middle temporal gyrus**.
The most inferior gyrus is the **inferior temporal gyrus**.

On the inferior side there are three gyri. Most medial of these is the **parahippocampal gyrus**, and next to it are the **medial** and **lateral occipitotemporal gyri** (that, as their names suggest, are continuous with the gyri of the same names in the occipital lobes).

Gyri of the parietal lobe

Like the frontal lobe, the parietal lobe also has a gyrus that runs next to and parallel to the central sulcus. Here, it is called the **postcentral gyrus**. Immediately behind it is the **postcentral sulcus**.

Posterior to it are the **superior** and **inferior parietal lobules**.

The inferior aspect of the inferior parietal lobule turns into two gyri:

The **supramarginal gyrus** encircles the posterior end of the lateral sulcus.
The **angular gyrus** lies posterior to the supramarginal gyrus.

Gyri of the occipital lobe

Comparing different sources, there does not seem to be a perfect agreement about what to call the gyri of the occipital lobes. One source even claims that the occipital lobe does not have any gyri with commonly used names. Thus, you should consider the following as an attempt to find some kind of consensus, but bear in mind that there probably is none.

The **cuneus** lies on the medial surface and above the lingual gyrus. Its anterior boundary is the **parietooccipital**

sulcus, and inferiorly its boundary is the **calcarine sulcus**.

The **lingual gyrus** lies on the inferior and medial side of the lobe. It then continues anteriorly as the parahippocampal gyrus.

On the inferior aspect, two gyri are found lateral to the lingual gyrus. They are called the **medial** and **lateral occipitotemporal gyri**; they continue into the temporal lobe.

Again, not only are the gyri rarely identical when different brains are compared, but they are also inconsistently named in different sources. Keep this in mind, and as always, use the names and definitions that your professors teach you.

Chapter 10

Cerebral Hemispheres (Sections)

The sagittal view

Suppose that we look at a sagittal section that shows the medial aspect of the right half of the brain, with the brainstem and cerebellum still attached to it.

The section shows the brainstem and the cerebellum with the fourth ventricle roughly between the pons and the cerebellum. It also shows the aqueduct connecting to the fourth ventricle from above.

If you follow the **aqueduct** from the fourth to the third ventricle, you find that it is leaning slightly in an anterior direction, and if you continue in that direction, you end up at a structure that exists in most but not all brains. It is the **interthalamic adhesion**, that connects the left and right thalamus. In a sagittal section, it is drawn as a small round shape. It is important that you identify it on the image, because the rest of the discussion relies on it.

Roughly anterior to it, there are two structures that are usually drawn in about the same size. First, you have the **interventricular foramen** (connecting the lateral ventricles to the third ventricle), and anterior to that, you have the **anterior commissure** (which, similar to the corpus callosum, allows crosstalk between the left and right hemispheres).

Between the interventricular foramen and the anterior commissure is the tip of a structure called the **fornix**. From the tip, it runs in a curved, superior and posterior direction, until it (in most drawings of this section) "disappears" into the corpus callosum.

Above the fornix is the large **corpus callosum**, and between them is the **septum pellucidum**, the thin wall that separates the left and right anterior horns of the lateral ventricle.

Inferior to the anterior commissure you find the three structures that, as you may remember from previous chapters, are encircled by the circle of Willis. They are, in anteroposterior direction, the **optic chiasma**, the **pituitary gland** (with its stalk, the **infundibulum**), and the **mammillary bodies**.

In about the same level in the posterior part of the midbrain, three structures are seen. Beginning inferiorly, they are the **inferior colliculi**, the **superior colliculi**, and the **pineal gland**.

The corpus callosum (as seen in a sagittal section)

In about the middle of the brain is this fairly large and white structure that connects the left and right hemispheres, called the **corpus callosum**.

Its main parts are the **rostrum**, **genu**, **body** and **splenium**. The body is the main central part, and the genu lies in front of it. The genu points anteriorly, bends down and then curves and points posteriorly, and this tapered, backward-pointing structure is called the rostrum. The splenium is the posterior part.

Above, and to some extent behind and below, the corpus callosum is a gyrus called the **cingulate gyrus**. And above (and, to some extent, behind and below) the cingulate gyrus is the **cingulate sulcus**.

The coronal view

Coronal sections demonstrate the diencephalon, basal ganglia, and other structures such as the hippocampus, the insula and the internal capsule most clearly.

Beginning at the superior midline, we see the **longitudinal fissure** separating the hemispheres.

At its most inferior limit, the longitudinal fissure has the **cingulate gyri** to its lateral sides, and below it is the **corpus callosum**.

Below the corpus callosum, the **lateral ventricles** on the sides and the **third ventricle** in the midline together form a shape that resembles the letter Y.

On both sides of the Y you find the left and right **thalamus**, whose medial sides are lateral to the third ventricle, and whose superior sides are inferior to the lateral ventricles.

Lateral to the thalamus is an important structure made up of white matter, known as the **internal capsule**.

Lateral to the internal capsule is the **lentiform nucleus**, which is a part of the **basal ganglia** (more on this later) and consists of the **globus pallidus** (most medial) and the **putamen** (most lateral). The globus pallidus is sometimes divided into a medial/internal and a lateral/external part.

Lateral to the lentiform nucleus is another white matter structure, called the **external capsule**.

Lateral to the external capsule is the long and thin (at least in a coronal section) **claustrum**.

Lateral to the claustrum is another white matter structure, called the **extreme capsule**.

Lateral to the extreme capsule is a part of the cerebral cortex called the **insula** (or the **insular cortex**).

Just like the cingulate gyri and the corpus callosum were found at the most inferior limit of the longitudinal fissure, the insula is found at the most medial limit of the lateral sulcus.

The cortical structures that form the walls of the lateral sulcus immediately lateral to the insula are together known as the **opercula**. These cortical structures come from the frontal, parietal and temporal lobes.

The **hippocampus** is found in the medial part of the temporal lobe where it "curls up" and takes a shape that with a little imagination resembles a sea horse (which has given the structure its name). It follows the floor of the inferior/temporal horn of the lateral ventricle (in the anteroposterior direction); below it is the parahippocampal gyrus.

Basal ganglia

One common definition of the **basal ganglia** is that they consist of these **four parts**: The **striatum**, the **globus pallidus**, the **substantia nigra**, and the **subthalamic nucleus**.

The **striatum**, in turn, consists of the **putamen** and the **caudate nucleus**. (The terminology is a jungle, but this definition of the striatum is a common one; be aware, though, that you might encounter other definitions.)

If you remember that the thalamus is lateral to the third ventricle and inferior to the lateral ventricle, understanding the course of the caudate nucleus will be easier.

The caudate nucleus is found essentially lateral to the thalamus, and roughly follows the "C-shape" that is suggested by the anterior/frontal and inferior/temporal horns of the lateral ventricle. (One way to remember this is to think of how eyeglass temples curve around the ear.)

The head of the caudate nucleus is wider, and lies more medial, than the tail.
(At the tip of the tail you find the **amygdala**.)

The **subthalamic nucleus** lies below the thalamus, and even further below, in the mesencephalon, is the **substantia nigra**, which contains cells that produce **dopamine**.

Corona radiata and internal capsule

The most superficial parts of the gyri and sulci of the cerebral cortex consist of **grey matter** (where the cell bodies of neurons are found), and below them is the **white matter** (that mostly contains myelinated axons of neurons).

The white matter in the superior parts of the cerebral hemispheres, closest to the grey matter, is called **centrum semiovale**.

Continuing downward, the white matter begins to look as if it is streaming towards or radiating from an inferior source. This "streaming" structure is known as the **corona radiata**.

The "inferior source" is the **internal capsule**, which thus is composed of bundles of axons carrying information to and from the cerebral cortex. It runs between the thalamus and the lentiform nucleus.

Multiple Choice Questions

These 150 multiple choice questions are composed based on the preceding text. Fifteen questions were created from each chapter, although in many cases, knowledge from many chapters will be required for understanding and solving the questions.

The questions are randomly arranged and come in chunks of ten, followed by the answers to the ten questions; thereafter, the next chunk of ten questions comes, and so on. I have chosen this arrangement so that you shouldn't have to flip back and forth all the time.

The choices that are given are most often either alphabetically or randomly arranged, so trying to solve the questions by searching for a secret pattern will not pay off. Also, I recommend that you try to think through not only why the correct answer is correct, but also why the false answers are false; actively thinking about the problem from many angles will boost your learning.

Some questions will probably be easy, and that is alright - it is actually reassuring, because it means that you already find critical and necessary information a piece of cake.

Good luck!

Questions 1-10

1:1
Looking at the brainstem dorsally, which round structure is found hanging in the midline superior to the superior colliculi?
1: Hypophysis
2: Hypothalamus
3: Mammillary body
4: Pineal gland

1:2
What is the most posterior part of the corpus callosum called?
1: Body
2: Genu
3: Operculum
4: Rostrum
5: Splenium

1:3
In the spinal cord, dorsal is the same as posterior, and ventral is the same as anterior. Which alternative describes the situation in the brain?
1: It is the same as in the spinal cord
2: It is the opposite as in the spinal cord
3: Dorsal is superior and ventral is inferior
4: Dorsal is inferior and ventral is superior

1:4
Which statement is true about the middle meningeal artery?
1: It enters through the foramen ovale and is implied in epidural hemorrhage
2: It enters through the foramen ovale and is implied in subdural hemorrhage

3: It enters through the foramen spinosum and is implied in epidural hemorrhage
4: It enters through the foramen spinosum and is implied in subdural hemorrhage

1:5
What are the names of the three lobes of the cerebellum?
1: Anterior, middle and posterior
2: Superior, middle and inferior
3: Anterior, posterior and flocculonodular
4: Superior, inferior and flocculonodular
5: Anterior, vermis and posterior
6: Superior, vermis and inferior

1:6
Which are the afferent and efferent limbs of the gag reflex?
1: Glossopharyngeal and hypoglossal, respectively
2: Hypoglossal and glossopharyngeal, respectively
3: Glossopharyngeal and vagal, respectively
4: Vagal and glossopharyngeal, respectively
5: Hypoglossal and vagal, respectively
6: Vagal and hypoglossal, respectively

1:7
In the neurocranium, four of the eight bones are two paired bones. Which two?
1: Ethmoid
2: Frontal
3: Occipital
4: Parietal
5: Sphenoid
6: Temporal

1:8
In which lobe of the cerebrum do you find the orbital gyri and sulci?
1: Frontal
2: Insula
3: Occipital
4: Parietal
5: Temporal

1:9
Which structures and in which order would a vibration signal from a limb travel through?
1: Contralateral dorsal column
2: Contralateral medial lemniscus
3: Contralateral spinal lemniscus
4: Ipsilateral dorsal column
5: Ipsilateral medial lemniscus
6: Ipsilateral spinal lemniscus

1:10
Which lobes do the anterior, posterior and inferior horns of the lateral ventricles reach into? State your answer in the right order.
1: Frontal
2: Occipital
3: Parietal
4: Temporal

Answers 1-10

1:1
Looking at the brainstem dorsally, which round structure is found hanging in the midline superior to the superior colliculi?
Answer: 4, pineal gland.

1:2
What is the most posterior part of the corpus callosum called?
Answer: 5, splenium.

1:3
In the spinal cord, dorsal is the same as posterior, and ventral is the same as anterior. Which alternative describes the situation in the brain?
Answer: 3, dorsal is superior and ventral is inferior.

1:4
Which statement is true about the middle meningeal artery?
Answer: 3, it enters through the foramen spinosum and is implied in epidural hemorrhage. The mandibular branch of the trigeminal nerve (V3) runs in the foramen ovale, and bridging veins are implied in subdural hemorrhage.

1:5
What are the names of the three lobes of the cerebellum?
Answer: 3, anterior, posterior and flocculonodular.

1:6
Which are the afferent and efferent limbs of the gag reflex?
Answer: 3, glossopharyngeal and vagal, respectively.

1:7

In the neurocranium, four of the eight bones are two paired bones. Which two?

Answer: 4 and 6, parietal and temporal.

1:8

In which lobe of the cerebrum do you find the orbital gyri and sulci?

Answer: 1, frontal lobe.

1:9

Which structures and in which order would a vibration signal from a limb travel through?

Answer: 4 and 2, ipsilateral dorsal column and contralateral medial lemniscus.

1:10

Which lobes do the anterior, posterior and inferior horns of the lateral ventricles reach into? State your answer in the right order.

Answer: 1, 2 and 4, frontal, occipital and temporal, respectively.

Questions 11-20

2:1

Which statement about the dorsal columns of the spinal cord is correct?
1: The dorsal columns continue in the brainstem as the medial lemniscus system
2: The signals that run in the dorsal columns decussate almost immediately after entering the spinal cord
3: The dorsal columns handle motor signals
4: The dorsal columns handle pain and temperature signals

2:2

What is included in the lentiform nucleus?
1: Globus pallidus, both external and internal parts
2: Putamen and globus pallidus
3: Putamen and caudate nucleus
4: Putamen, globus pallidus and caudate nucleus

2:3

Which statement about the facial nerve's exit point from the brainstem is true?
1: It leaves from the posterior pons
2: It leaves in the ventrolateral sulcus in the medulla oblongata
3: It leaves in the dorsolateral sulcus in the medulla oblongata
4: It leaves laterally between the pons and the medulla oblongata
5: It leaves medially between the pons and the medulla oblongata

2:4

Which of these are the two names used for the widening
or groove that separates the temporal lobe from the
frontal and parietal lobes?
1: Central sulcus
2: Lateral sulcus
3: Longitudinal fissure
4: Rolandic fissure
5: Sylvian fissure

2:5

Place the four deep cerebellar nuclei in medial to lateral
order.
1: Dentate nucleus
2: Emboliform nucleus
3: Fastigial nucleus
4: Globose nucleus

2:6

From which structure or structures do the median and
lateral apertures extend?
1: All three apertures from the lateral ventricles
2: All three apertures from the third ventricle
3: All three apertures from the fourth ventricle
4: Median aperture from third ventricle, lateral apertures
from lateral ventricles
5: Median aperture from fourth ventricle, lateral apertures
from lateral ventricles

2:7

Which of these vessels, and in which order, would blood
from the aorta normally pass before it arrived in the left
anterior cerebral artery?
1: Anterior communicating artery
2: Basilar artery
3: Brachiocephalic trunk

4: Left common carotid artery
5: Left external carotid artery
6: Left internal carotid artery
7: Left subclavian artery
8: Left vertebral artery

2:8
An upwards movement between two points in the spinal cord can be described with either of which two terms?
1: Rostral and anterior
2: Rostral and caudal
3: Rostral and cranial
4: Rostral and dorsal

2:9
Which two structures do not travel through the jugular foramen?
1: Glossopharyngeal nerve
2: Vagus nerve
3: Accessory nerve
4: Hypoglossal nerve
5: External jugular vein
6: Internal jugular vein

2:10
Which of these structures are found in the mesencephalon? More than one alternative may be correct.
1: Cerebral peduncle
2: Crus cerebri
3: Globose nucleus
4: Red nucleus
5: Substantia nigra

Answers 11-20

2:1
Which statement about the dorsal columns of the spinal cord is correct?
Answer: 1, the dorsal columns continue in the brainstem as the medial lemniscus system.

2:2
What is included in the lentiform nucleus?
Answer: 2, putamen and globus pallidus.

2:3
Which statement about the facial nerve's exit point from the brainstem is true?
Answer: 4, it leaves laterally between the pons and the medulla oblongata.

2:4
Which of these are the two names used for the widening or groove that separates the temporal lobe from the frontal and parietal lobes?
Answer: 2 and 5, lateral sulcus and Sylvian fissure.

2:5
Place the four deep cerebellar nuclei in medial to lateral order.
Answer: 3, 4, 2 and 1, fastigial, globose, emboliform and dentate.

2:6
From which structure or structures do the median and lateral apertures extend?
Answer: 3, all three apertures extend from the fourth ventricle.

2:7
Which of these vessels, and in which order, would blood from the aorta normally pass before it arrived in the left anterior cerebral artery?
Answer: 4 and 6, left common carotid artery and left internal carotid artery.

2:8
An upwards movement between two points in the spinal cord can be described with either of which two terms?
Answer: 3, rostral and cranial.

2:9
Which two structures do not travel through the jugular foramen?
Answer: 4 and 5, the hypoglossal nerve (which travels through the hypoglossal canal) and the external jugular vein (which is not found inside the cranium).

2:10
Which of these structures are found in the mesencephalon? More than one alternative may be correct.
Answer: 1, 2, 4 and 5, the cerebral peduncles, crus cerebri, red nucleus and substantia nigra are found in the mesencephalon.

Questions 21-30

3:1
Which two statements are true about the oculomotor and trochlear nerves?
1: They both leave from the anterior side of the brainstem
2: They both leave from the posterior side of the brainstem
3: They both leave the cranium through the optic canal
4: They both leave the cranium through the superior orbital fissure
5: The oculomotor nerve's nuclei lie caudal to the trochlear nerve's nuclei
6: The trochlear nerve's nuclei lie caudal to the oculomotor nerve's nuclei

3:2
Which important substances are produced by the substantia nigra and locus coeruleus, respectively?
1: Dopamine and epinephrine, respectively
2: Dopamine and norepinephrine, respectively
3: Epinephrine and dopamine, respectively
4: Epinephrine and norepinephrine, respectively
5: Norepinephrine and dopamine, respectively
6: Norepinephrine and epinephrine, respectively

3:3
Out of which embryological structure does the third ventricle arise?
1: Telencephalon
2: Diencephalon
3: Mesencephalon
4: Metencephalon
5: Myelencephalon

3:4
What is the name of the fissure that separates the posterior lobe from the flocculonodular lobe in the cerebellum?
1: Horizontal fissure
2: Posterolateral fissure
3: Primary fissure
4: Secondary fissure

3:5
The external capsule runs between which two structures?
1: Thalamus and globus pallidus
2: Globus pallidus and putamen
3: Putamen and claustrum
4: Claustrum and insula

3:6
Which statement is true about the anterior inferior cerebellar artery (AICA) and the superior cerebellar artery (SCA)?
1: Both are branches of the vertebral arteries
2: Both are branches of the basilar artery
3: AICA is a branch of the vertebral artery, SCA of the basilar artery
4: SCA is a branch of the vertebral artery, AICA of the basilar artery

3:7
There is a smaller lobe within the occipital lobe, that is found between the parietooccipital and calcarine sulci. What is its name?
1: Cingulate gyrus
2: Cuneus
3: Lingual gyrus
4: Orbital gyri
5: Uncus

3:8
Which statement about the spinal cord is correct?
1: The bundle of nerves that hang down within the lower part of the vertebral column is called the filum terminale
2: The tapered lower end of the spinal cord is called the cauda equina
3: The part of the spinal cord that is found immediately below the brainstem is called the conus medullaris
4: The spinal cord is surrounded by the same three meningeal layers (pia/arachnoid/dura mater) as the brain

3:9
Which three cranial bones form the anterior cranial fossa?
1: Ethmoid bone
2: Frontal bone
3: Occipital bone
4: Parietal bone
5: Sphenoid bone
6: Temporal bone

3:10
When discussing the cerebrum, which alternative is a synonym to superior?
1: Anterior
2: Dorsal
3: Posterior
4: Ventral

Answers 21-30

3:1
Which two statements are true about the oculomotor and trochlear nerves?
Answer: 4 and 6, they both leave the cranium through the superior orbital fissure, and the trochlear nerve's nuclei lie caudal to the oculomotor nerve's nuclei.

3:2
Which important substances are produced by the substantia nigra and locus coeruleus, respectively?
Answer: 2, dopamine and norepinephrine, respectively.

3:3
Out of which embryological structure does the third ventricle arise?
Answer: 2, diencephalon gives rise to the third ventricle.

3:4
What is the name of the fissure that separates the posterior lobe from the flocculonodular lobe in the cerebellum?
Answer: 2, posterolateral fissure.

3:5
The external capsule runs between which two structures?
Answer: 3, putamen and claustrum.

3:6
Which statement is true about the anterior inferior cerebellar artery (AICA) and the superior cerebellar artery (SCA)?
Answer: 2, both are branches of the basilar artery.

3:7
There is a smaller lobe within the occipital lobe, that is found between the parietooccipital and calcarine sulci. What is its name?
Answer: 2, cuneus.

3:8
Which statement about the spinal cord is correct?
Answer: 4, the spinal cord is surrounded by the same three meningeal layers (pia/arachnoid/dura mater) as the brain.

3:9
Which three cranial bones form the anterior cranial fossa?
Answer: 1, 2 and 5, the ethmoid, frontal and sphenoid bones.

3:10
When discussing the cerebrum, which alternative is a synonym to superior?
Answer: 2, dorsal.

Questions 31-40

4:1
Where in the cerebrum do you find the supramarginal gyrus?
1: Frontal lobe
2: Occipital lobe
3: Parietal lobe
4: Temporal lobe

4:2
What are the names of cranial nerves VIII and IX?
1: Abducens
2: Facial
3: Glossopharyngeal
4: Vagus
5: Vestibulocochlear

4:3
Which artery serves the medial parts of the frontal lobes?
1: Anterior cerebral artery
2: Anterior communicating artery
3: Middle cerebral artery
4: Middle meningeal artery

4:4
What is the name given to the combination of the putamen and the caudate nucleus?
1: Globus pallidus
2: Interposed nuclei
3: Lentiform nucleus
4: Striatum

4:5
In the medulla oblongata, what is the groove between the pyramid and the olive called?
1: Anterior median fissure
2: Dorsolateral sulcus
3: Posterior median sulcus
4: Ventrolateral sulcus

4:6
Moving from the tectum to the tegmentum in the mesencephalon - which of the alternatives describes the movement most accurately?
1: Anterior to posterior
2: Caudal to rostral
3: Lateral to medial
4: Medial to lateral
5: Posterior to anterior
6: Rostral to caudal

4:7
What is another name for the interventricular foramina between the lateral and third ventricles?
1: Foramina of Magendie
2: Foramina of Monro
3: Foramina of Luschka
4: Foramina of Sylvius

4:8
The surface of the cerebellum has many thin ridges. What are they called?
1: Folia
2: Gyri
3: Lobules
4: Sulci

4:9
Which tract in the spinal cord carries proprioceptive signals from the right leg?
1: Left fasciculus cuneatus
2: Left fasciculus gracilis
3: Right fasciculus cuneatus
4: Right fasciculus gracilis

4:10
What passes the cavernous sinus but not the superior orbital fissure? More than one answer could be correct.
1: Internal carotid artery
2: Oculomotor nerve
3: Trochlear nerve
4: Trigeminal nerve, branch V1
5: Trigeminal nerve, branch V2
6: Trigeminal nerve, branch V3
7: Abducens nerve

Answers 31-40

4:1
Where in the cerebrum do you find the supramarginal gyrus?
Answer: 3, parietal lobe.

4:2
What are the names of cranial nerves VIII and IX?
Answer: 5 and 3, vestibulocochlear and glossopharyngeal.

4:3
Which artery serves the medial parts of the frontal lobes?
Answer: 1, anterior cerebral artery.

4:4
What is the name given to the combination of the putamen and the caudate nucleus?
Answer: 4, striatum.

4:5
In the medulla oblongata, what is the groove between the pyramid and the olive called?
Answer: 4, ventrolateral sulcus (or anterolateral sulcus, or pre-olivary sulcus).

4:6
Moving from the tectum to the tegmentum in the mesencephalon - which of the alternatives describes the movement most accurately?
Answer: 5, posterior to anterior.

4:7
What is another name for the interventricular foramina between the lateral and third ventricles?
Answer: 2, foramina of Monro.

4:8
The surface of the cerebellum has many thin ridges. What are they called?
Answer: 1, folia.

4:9
Which tract in the spinal cord carries proprioceptive signals from the right leg?
Answer: 4, right fasciculus gracilis.

4:10
What passes the cavernous sinus but not the superior orbital fissure? More than one answer could be correct.
Answer: 1 and 5, the internal carotid artery and the maxillary branch of the trigeminal nerve (V2). The ophthalmic branch of the trigeminal nerve (V1) and the oculomotor, trochlear and abducens nerves all pass through both structures, while the mandibular branch of the trigeminal nerve (V3) passes through neither.

Questions 41-50

5:1
Which statement is false about the cerebellum?
1: The middle cerebellar peduncles connect the cerebellum to the midbrain
2: The primary fissure separates the anterior and posterior lobes
3: The horizontal fissure is found in the posterior lobe
4: The vermis is included in the term spinocerebellum

5:2
Which two cranial nerves send taste impulses from the tongue to the central nervous system?
1: Facial nerve
2: Glossopharyngeal nerve
3: Hypoglossal nerve
4: Trigeminal nerve

5:3
What is the name given to the combination of the putamen and the globus pallidus?
1: Caudate nucleus
2: Interposed nuclei
3: Lentiform nucleus
4: Striatum

5:4
When discussing the cerebrum, which alternative is a synonym to ventral?
1: Back part
2: Frontal part
3: Lower part
4: Upper part

5:5
Which tract in the spinal cord carries proprioceptive signals from the left arm?
1: Left fasciculus cuneatus
2: Left fasciculus gracilis
3: Right fasciculus cuneatus
4: Right fasciculus gracilis

5:6
Which two statements are correct?
1: The vertebral arteries enter the cranium through the foramen magnum
2: The right internal carotid artery is a branch of the brachiocephalic trunk
3: The right vertebral artery is a branch of the right subclavian artery
4: The right internal carotid artery is a branch of the right subclavian artery
5: The vertebral arteries are part of the anterior circulation

5:7
Which two structures travel through the foramen ovale and the foramen rotundum? State your answers in the correct order.
1: CN V, V1
2: CN V, V2
3: CN V, V3
4: Middle meningeal artery

5:8
Where in the cerebrum do you find the calcarine sulcus?
1: Frontal lobe
2: Occipital lobe
3: Parietal lobe
4: Temporal lobe

5:9
Two cranial nerves exit the brainstem at the cerebello-pontine angle. Which ones?
1: Abducens nerve
2: Facial nerve
3: Glossopharyngeal nerve
4: Trigeminal nerve
5: Trochlear nerve
6: Vestibulocochlear nerve

5:10
Through which structure is cerebrospinal fluid drained into the blood circulation?
1: Arachnoid granulations
2: Choroid plexus
3: Median aperture
4: Lateral apertures

Answers 41-50

5:1
Which statement is false about the cerebellum?
Answer: 1, the middle cerebellar peduncles connect the cerebellum to the midbrain.

5:2
Which two cranial nerves send taste impulses from the tongue to the central nervous system?
Answer: 1 and 2, the facial and glossopharyngeal nerves.

5:3
What is the name given to the combination of the putamen and the globus pallidus?
Answer: 3, lentiform nucleus.

5:4
When discussing the cerebrum, which alternative is a synonym to ventral?
Answer: 3, lower part.

5:5
Which tract in the spinal cord carries proprioceptive signals from the left arm?
Answer: 1, left fasciculus cuneatus.

5:6
Which two statements are correct?
Answer: 1 and 3, the vertebral arteries enter the cranium through the foramen magnum, and both of them are branches of the subclavian arteries. The right internal carotid artery is a branch of the right common carotid artery, which, however, is a branch of the brachiocephalic trunk. The vertebral arteries are part of the posterior circulation.

5:7

Which two structures travel through the foramen ovale and the foramen rotundum? State your answers in the correct order.

Answer: 3 and 2 (mandibular and maxillary branches of the trigeminal nerve, respectively). The ophthalmic branch (V1) of the trigeminal nerve travels through the superior orbital fissure, and the middle meningeal artery travels through the foramen spinosum.

5:8

Where in the cerebrum do you find the calcarine sulcus?
Answer: 2, occipital lobe.

5:9

Two cranial nerves exit the brainstem at the cerebello-pontine angle. Which ones?
Answer: 2 and 6, facial and vestibulocochlear nerves.

5:10

Through which structure is cerebrospinal fluid drained into the blood circulation?
Answer: 1, arachnoid granulations.

Questions 51-60

6:1
What travels in the spinal lemniscus in the brainstem?
1: Ascending motor signals
2: Ascending pain and temperature signals
3: Ascending proprioception signals
4: Descending motor signals
5: Descending pain and temperature signals
6: Descending proprioception signals

6:2
Which of the cranial bones does the sella turcica arise from?
1: Ethmoid bone
2: Frontal bone
3: Occipital bone
4: Parietal bone
5: Sphenoid bone
6: Temporal bone

6:3
Venous blood flows from the confluence of sinuses to the transverse sinus. Which are the three major direct contributors to the confluence?
1: Inferior sagittal sinus, superior sagittal sinus and occipital sinus
2: Inferior sagittal sinus, superior sagittal sinus and straight sinus
3: Inferior sagittal sinus, occipital sinus and straight sinus
4: Superior sagittal sinus, occipital sinus and straight sinus

6:4
What is the name of the fissure that separates the anterior lobe from the posterior lobe in the cerebellum?
1: Horizontal fissure
2: Posterolateral fissure
3: Primary fissure
4: Secondary fissure

6:5
On the medial side of the frontal lobe, which structure lies immediately inferior to the structure called medial frontal gyrus in some sources and superior frontal gyrus in others?
1: Cingulate gyrus
2: Cingulate sulcus
3: Inferior frontal gyrus
4: Medial prefrontal gyrus
5: Middle frontal gyrus

6:6
Which statement is true?
1: The cerebral peduncles are posterior to the substantia nigra
2: The aqueduct is caudal to the central canal
3: The olives are anterior to the pyramids
4: The superior colliculi are posterior to the aqueduct

6:7
What is the point at which the fourth ventricle narrows and turns into the central canal in the medulla oblongata called?
1: Choroid plexus
2: Cistern
3: Fornix
4: Obex

6:8
If you injure the entire left side of your spinal cord at a level that would give you symptoms from the lower extremity, what would be the expected symptoms?
1: Loss of pain and vibration in the left leg
2: Loss of pain and vibration in the right leg
3: Loss of pain in the left leg, loss of vibration in the right leg
4: Loss of pain in the right leg, loss of vibration in the left leg

6:9
What is the name of the gyri found immediately lateral to the most inferior limit of the longitudinal fissure?
1: Cingulate gyri
2: Inferior frontal gyri
3: Insula
4: Medial frontal gyri
5: Middle frontal gyri

6:10
The cranial nerves that control the movement of the eyes are CN III, IV and VI. What are their corresponding names?
1: Abducens, oculomotor, trochlear
2: Abducens, trochlear, oculomotor
3: Oculomotor, abducens, trochlear
4: Oculomotor, trochlear, abducens
5: Trochlear, abducens, oculomotor
6: Trochlear, oculomotor, abducens

Answers 51-60

6:1
What travels in the spinal lemniscus in the brainstem?
Answer: 2, ascending pain and temperature signals.

6:2
Which of the cranial bones does the sella turcica arise from?
Answer: 5, sphenoid bone.

6:3
Venous blood flows from the confluence of sinuses to the transverse sinus. Which are the three major direct contributors to the confluence?
Answer: 4, superior sagittal sinus, occipital sinus and straight sinus. The inferior sagittal sinus drains into the straight sinus and is therefore not a direct contributor.

6:4
What is the name of the fissure that separates the anterior lobe from the posterior lobe in the cerebellum?
Answer: 3, primary fissure.

6:5
On the medial side of the frontal lobe, which structure lies immediately inferior to the structure called medial frontal gyrus in some sources and superior frontal gyrus in others?
Answer: 2, cingulate sulcus.

6:6
Which statement is true?
Answer: 4, the superior colliculi are posterior to the aqueduct.

6:7
What is the point at which the fourth ventricle narrows
and turns into the central canal in the medulla oblongata
called?
Answer: 4, obex.

6:8
If you injure the entire left side of your spinal cord at a
level that would give you symptoms from the lower extremity, what would be the expected symptoms?
Answer: 4, loss of pain in the right leg (fibers decussate
almost immediately) and loss of vibration in the left leg
(fibers decussate in the level of the pyramid in the
medulla oblongata).

6:9
What is the name of the gyri found immediately lateral to
the most inferior limit of the longitudinal fissure?
Answer: 1, cingulate gyri.

6:10
The cranial nerves that control the movement of the eyes
are CN III, IV and VI. What are their corresponding
names?
Answer: 4, oculomotor, trochlear and abducens.

Questions 61-70

7:1
Where is the locus coeruleus found?
1: Caudal, dorsal pons
2: Caudal, ventral pons
3: Rostral, dorsal pons
4: Rostral, ventral pons

7:2
Which two structures are separating the cerebral hemi-spheres from each other and the frontal and parietal lobes, respectively?
1: Central sulcus and lateral sulcus
2: Lateral sulcus and central sulcus
3: Central sulcus and longitudinal fissure
4: Longitudinal fissure and central sulcus
5: Lateral sulcus and longitudinal fissure
6: Longitudinal fissure and lateral sulcus

7:3
Between which two arteries does the posterior communi-cating artery run?
1: Basilar artery and posterior cerebral artery
2: Left and right posterior cerebral arteries
3: Posterior cerebral artery and anterior cerebral artery
4: Posterior cerebral artery and internal carotid artery
5: Posterior cerebral artery and middle cerebral artery

7:4
Which term best describes the position of the foramen magnum in relation to the sella turcica?
1: Anterior
2: Lateral
3: Medial
4: Posterior

7:5
What is included in the striatum?
1: Globus pallidus, both external and internal parts
2: Putamen and globus pallidus
3: Putamen and caudate nucleus
4: Putamen, globus pallidus and caudate nucleus

7:6
Which statement is correct about the arrangement in the spinal cord?
1: The fasciculus gracilis is lateral to the fasciculus cuneatus
2: The lateral corticospinal tract is posterior to the lateral spinothalamic tract
3: The anterior corticospinal tract is lateral to the anterior spinothalamic tract
4: The spinocerebellar tracts lie close to the midline

7:7
What is the space between the dura mater and bone called?
1: Epidural space
2: Extracranial space
3: Intradural space
4: Subarachnoidal space
5: Subdural space

7:8
Which of these extraocular muscles is not innervated by the oculomotor nerve?
1: Inferior oblique
2: Inferior rectus
3: Medial rectus
4: Superior oblique
5: Superior rectus

7:9
Which structure runs through the third ventricle?
1: Anterior commissure
2: Central canal
3: Interthalamic adhesion
4: Median aperture

7:10
Which statement is true about the cerebellum?
1: The emboliform nuclei are found in the cerebellar white matter
2: Arbor vitae is Latin for "white matter"
3: The vermis runs along the horizontal fissure
4: The falx cerebri dips into the cerebellum and separates the left and right hemispheres

Answers 61-70

7:1
Where is the locus coeruleus found?
Answer: 3, rostral, dorsal pons.

7:2
Which two structures are separating the cerebral hemispheres from each other and the frontal and parietal
lobes, respectively?
Answer: 4, longitudinal fissure and central sulcus.

7:3
Between which two arteries does the posterior communicating artery run?
Answer: 4, posterior cerebral artery and internal carotid
artery.

7:4
Which term best describes the position of the foramen
magnum in relation to the sella turcica?
Answer: 4, posterior.

7:5
What is included in the striatum?
Answer: 3, putamen and caudate nucleus.

7:6
Which statement is correct about the arrangement in the
spinal cord?
Answer: 2, the lateral corticospinal tract is posterior to
the lateral spinothalamic tract.

7:7

What is the space between the dura mater and bone called?

Answer: 1, epidural space.

7:8

Which of these extraocular muscles is not innervated by the oculomotor nerve?

Answer: 4, superior oblique (this is innervated by the trochlear nerve).

7:9

Which structure runs through the third ventricle?

Answer: 3, interthalamic adhesion (although, as mentioned in the text, it is sometimes absent).

7:10

Which statement is true about the cerebellum?

Answer: 1, the emboliform nuclei are found in the cerebellar white matter. Arbor vitae is Latin for "tree of life," and the vermis runs perpendicular to the horizontal fissure. The falx cerebri does not dip into the cerebellum at all.

Questions 71-80

8:1
Which structure within the ventricular system is producing the cerebrospinal fluid?
1: Arachnoid granulations
2: Choroid plexus
3: Fornix
4: Obex
5: Septum pellucidum

8:2
Which structure is found between the crura cerebri and tegmentum of the mesencephalon?
1: Cerebral peduncle
2: Obex
3: Substantia nigra
4: Tectum

8:3
Which structure is found below the floor of the temporal horn of the lateral ventricle?
1: Amygdala
2: Insula
3: Cingulate gyrus
4: Hippocampus
5: Hypothalamus

8:4
Which are the afferent and efferent limbs of the corneal reflex?
1: CN II and CN III, respectively
2: CN II and CN VII, respectively
3: CN V and CN III, respectively
4: CN V and CN VII, respectively

8:5
Which term best describes the position of the putamen in relation to the claustrum?
1: Anterior
2: Inferior
3: Lateral
4: Medial
5: Posterior
6: Superior

8:6
Which of the cranial bones do the crista galli and cribriform plate arise from?
1: Ethmoid bone
2: Frontal bone
3: Occipital bone
4: Parietal bone
5: Sphenoid bone
6: Temporal bone

8:7
In the medial and inferior parts of the cerebellum's posterior lobe, close to the foramen magnum, there are two bulging structures. What are they called?
1: Folia
2: Inferior cerebellar peduncles
3: Medial cerebellar peduncles
4: Tonsils
5: Vermis

8:8
Which are the two major contributors to the straight sinus?
1: Great cerebral vein (of Galen) and inferior sagittal sinus
2: Great cerebral vein (of Galen) and superior sagittal sinus

3: Transverse sinus and inferior sagittal sinus
4: Transverse sinus and superior sagittal sinus

8:9
Which of these tracts do not decussate at the level of the medulla oblongata? More than one answer may be correct.
1: Anterior corticospinal tract
2: Anterior spinothalamic tract
3: Lateral corticospinal tract
4: Lateral spinothalamic tract

8:10
What is the name of the gyrus that lies immediately in front of the sulcus that separates the frontal and parietal lobes?
1: Precentral gyrus
2: Prefrontal gyrus
3: Postcentral gyrus
4: Postfrontal gyrus

Answers 71-80

8:1
Which structure within the ventricular system is producing the cerebrospinal fluid?
Answer: 2, choroid plexus.

8:2
Which structure is found between the crura cerebri and tegmentum of the mesencephalon?
Answer: 3, substantia nigra.

8:3
Which structure is found below the floor of the temporal horn of the lateral ventricle?
Answer: 4, hippocampus.

8:4
Which are the afferent and efferent limbs of the corneal reflex?
Answer: 4, CN V and CN VII (trigeminal and facial), respectively.

8:5
Which term best describes the position of the putamen in relation to the claustrum?
Answer: 4, medial.

8:6
Which of the cranial bones do the crista galli and cribriform plate arise from?
Answer: 1, ethmoid bone.

8:7
In the medial and inferior parts of the cerebellum's posterior lobe, close to the foramen magnum, there are two

bulging structures. What are they called?
Answer: 4, tonsils.

8:8
Which are the two major contributors to the straight sinus?
Answer: 1, great cerebral vein and inferior sagittal sinus.

8:9
Which of these tracts do not decussate at the level of the medulla oblongata? More than one answer may be correct.
Answer: 1, 2 and 4.

8:10
What is the name of the gyrus that lies immediately in front of the sulcus that separates the frontal and parietal lobes?
Answer: 1, precentral gyrus.

Questions 81-90

9:1
Which tract in the spinal cord carries pain signals from the right leg?
1: Left dorsal column
2: Right dorsal column
3: Left spinothalamic tract
4: Right spinothalamic tract

9:2
What is the name of the gyrus that lies immediately behind the sulcus that separates the frontal and parietal lobes?
1: Precentral gyrus
2: Prefrontal gyrus
3: Postcentral gyrus
4: Postfrontal gyrus

9:3
Which statement is true about the cerebellum?
1: The horizontal fissure divides the cerebellum into the two hemispheres
2: The anterior lobe consists of the three most anterior lobules
3: The posterior lobe consists of the five most posterior lobules
4: The vermis marks the division between the anterior and posterior lobes

9:4
Moving from the pons to the mesencephalon - which of the alternatives describes the movement most accurately?
1: Anterior to posterior
2: Caudal to rostral

3: Lateral to medial
4: Medial to lateral
5: Posterior to anterior
6: Rostral to caudal

9:5
From which artery does the posterior inferior cerebellar artery branch off?
1: Vertebral artery
2: Basilar artery
3: Posterior cerebral artery
4: Posterior communicating artery
5: Internal carotid artery

9:6
Which cranial nerve is the recurrent nerve a branch of?
1: Accessory (cranial part)
2: Accessory (spinal part)
3: Glossopharyngeal
4: Trochlear
5: Vagus

9:7
The internal capsule runs between which two structures?
1: Thalamus and globus pallidus
2: Globus pallidus and putamen
3: Putamen and claustrum
4: Claustrum and insula

9:8
What is the name of the suture that connects the parietal and temporal bones of the neurocranium?
1: Coronal suture
2: Lambdoid suture
3: Sagittal suture
4: Squamosal suture

9:9
Which part of the ventricular system arises from the embryological structure called mesencephalon?
1: Lateral ventricles
2: Foramina of Monro
3: Third ventricle
4: Aqueduct of Sylvius
5: Fourth ventricle

9:10
Which structure is separated from the olive by the dorsolateral sulcus in the medulla oblongata?
1: Inferior cerebellar peduncle
2: Obex
3: Pyramid
4: Tectum

Answers 81-90

9:1
Which tract in the spinal cord carries pain signals from the right leg?
Answer: 3, left spinothalamic tract.

9:2
What is the name of the gyrus that lies immediately behind the sulcus that separates the frontal and parietal lobes?
Answer: 3, postcentral gyrus

9:3
Which statement is true about the cerebellum?
Answer: 2, the anterior lobe consists of the three most anterior lobules.

9:4
Moving from the pons to the mesencephalon - which of the alternatives describes the movement most accurately?
Answer: 2, caudal to rostral.

9:5
From which artery does the posterior inferior cerebellar artery branch off?
Answer: 1, vertebral artery.

9:6
Which cranial nerve is the recurrent nerve a branch of?
Answer: 5, vagus.

9:7
The internal capsule runs between which two structures?
Answer: 1, thalamus and globus pallidus.

9:8
What is the name of the suture that connects the parietal and temporal bones of the neurocranium?
Answer: 4, squamosal suture.

9:9
Which part of the ventricular system arises from the embryological structure called mesencephalon?
Answer: 4, aqueduct of Sylvius.

9:10
Which structure is separated from the olive by the dorsolateral sulcus in the medulla oblongata?
Answer: 1, inferior cerebellar peduncle.

Questions 91-100

10:1
Which of these are the three main branches of the trigeminal nerve (V1, V2 and V3)?
1: Mandibular
2: Maxillary
3: Nasal
4: Temporal
5: Ophthalmic

10:2
Which of the three germ layers does the nervous system originate from?
1: Ectoderm
2: Endoderm
3: Mesoderm

10:3
What dominates the content in the crura cerebri of the mesencephalon?
1: Ascending motor signals
2: Ascending pain and temperature signals
3: Ascending proprioception signals
4: Descending motor signals
5: Descending pain and temperature signals
6: Descending proprioception signals

10:4
What is separating the anterior horns of the left and right lateral ventricles from each other?
1: Choroid plexus
2: Interventricular foramina
3: Median aperture
4: Septum pellucidum

10:5
What is found immediately below the lateral sulcus of the cerebrum?
1: Inferior parietal lobule
2: Inferior temporal gyrus
3: Superior parietal lobule
4: Superior temporal gyrus

10:6
Which structures and in which order would a pain signal from a limb travel through?
1: Contralateral dorsal column
2: Contralateral spinothalamic tract
3: Dorsal root
4: Ipsilateral dorsal column
5: Ipsilateral spinothalamic tract
6: Ventral root

10:7
What is true about the blood supply of the spinal cord?
1: There is one posterior spinal artery that runs along the midline and gets reinforced throughout its path down to the caudal spinal cord
2: The arteries of Adamkiewicz branch off from the posterior inferior cerebellar arteries and form the anterior spinal artery
3: The two posterior spinal arteries are branches of the common carotid arteries
4: Two medial branches from the vertebral arteries meet in the anterior midline and form the anterior spinal artery

10:8
The cortical walls immediately lateral to the insular cortex, within the lateral sulcus, are called what?
1: Cingulate gyrus
2: Claustrum

3: Orbital gyri
4: Opercula

10:9
What is included in the term "leptomeninges"?
1: Arachnoid and dura mater
2: Arachnoid and pia mater
3: Dura mater and pia mater
4: Dura, arachnoid and pia mater

10:10
Which is the only true statement about the cerebellum?
1: The inferior cerebellar peduncles connect the cerebellum to the medulla oblongata
2: The cerebral peduncles connect the cerebellum to the cerebrum
3: The left and right cerebellar hemispheres are divided by a fold of the dura mater called tentorium cerebelli
4: The middle cerebellar peduncle attaches to the midbrain

Answers 91-100

10:1
Which of these are the three main branches of the trigeminal nerve (V1, V2 and V3)?
Answer: 5, 2 and 1 (ophthalmic, maxillary, mandibular).

10:2
Which of the three germ layers does the nervous system originate from?
Answer: 1, ectoderm.

10:3
What dominates the content in the crura cerebri of the mesencephalon?
Answer: 4, descending motor signals.

10:4
What is separating the anterior horns of the left and right lateral ventricles from each other?
Answer: 4, septum pellucidum.

10:5
What is found immediately below the lateral sulcus of the cerebrum?
Answer: 4, superior temporal gyrus.

10:6
Which structures and in which order would a pain signal from a limb travel through?
Answer: 3 and 2, dorsal root and contralateral spinothalamic tract.

10:7
What is true about the blood supply of the spinal cord?
Answer: 4, two medial branches from the vertebral arter-

ies meet in the anterior midline and form the anterior spinal artery.

10:8
The cortical walls immediately lateral to the insular cortex, within the lateral sulcus, are called what?
Answer: 4, opercula.

10:9
What is included in the term "leptomeninges"?
Answer: 2, arachnoid and pia mater.

10:10
Which is the only true statement about the cerebellum?
Answer: 1, the inferior cerebellar peduncles connect the cerebellum to the medulla oblongata.

Questions 101-110

11:1
What lies immediately anterior to the postcentral sulcus of the cerebrum?
1: Central sulcus
2: Postcentral gyrus
3: Precentral gyrus
4: Precentral sulcus

11:2
Which of these vessels, and in which order, would blood from the brachiocephalic trunk normally pass before it arrived in the anterior inferior cerebellar artery?
1: Basilar artery
2: Left common carotid artery
3: Right common carotid artery
4: Left subclavian artery
5: Right subclavian artery
6: Left vertebral artery
7: Right vertebral artery
8: Posterior cerebral artery

11:3
What is the structure found in the midline of the cerebellum, between the two hemispheres, called?
1: Flocculus
2: Folia
3: Nodule
4: Tonsil
5: Vermis

11:4
The supratentorial and infratentorial compartments are separated by which structure?
1: Falx cerebelli

2: Falx cerebri
3: Foramen magnum
4: Tentorium cerebelli

11:5
Which cranial nerve do you see below the inferior colliculi?
1: Abducens nerve
2: Oculomotor nerve
3: Optic nerve
4: Trochlear nerve

11:6
Which statement is true?
1: The globus pallidus is lateral to the thalamus
2: The putamen is medial to the globus pallidus
3: The thalamus is lateral to the internal capsule
4: The claustrum is medial to the external capsule

11:7
Which of the following is not a fold of the dura mater?
1: Diaphragma sellae
2: Falx cerebelli
3: Falx cerebri
4: Septum pellucidum
5: Tentorium cerebelli

11:8
Which statement about the spinal cord is correct?
1: The ventral and dorsal horns join and form the spinal nerves
2: The dorsal roots carry efferent signals into the spinal cord
3: The dorsal root ganglia lie outside of the spinal cord
4: In some parts of the spinal cord, the white matter bulges out to the sides and forms lateral horns

11:9
Which statement is correct?
1: Visual signals from the retina enter the thalamus before the optic chiasma
2: Visual signals from the lateral part of the right retina pass the right thalamus
3: Visual signals from the left side of the visual field split up in the optic chiasma and are sent to both the left and right occipital lobes
4: After leaving the thalamus, the signals are transferred to the occipital cortex via the optic tract

11:10
Which structure connects the third and fourth ventricles?
1: Aqueduct of Sylvius
2: Central canal
3: Lateral apertures
4: Median aperture
5: Septum pellucidum

Answers 101-110

11:1
What lies immediately anterior to the postcentral sulcus of the cerebrum?
Answer: 2, postcentral gyrus.

11:2
Which of these vessels, and in which order, would blood from the brachiocephalic trunk normally pass before it arrived in the anterior inferior cerebellar artery?
Answer: 5, 7 and 1, right subclavian artery, right vertebral artery and basilar artery.

11:3
What is the structure found in the midline of the cerebellum, between the two hemispheres, called?
Answer: 5, vermis.

11:4
The supratentorial and infratentorial compartments are separated by which structure?
Answer: 4, tentorium cerebelli.

11:5
Which cranial nerve do you see below the inferior colliculi?
Answer: 4, trochlear nerve (the only cranial nerve that exits from the dorsal side of the brainstem).

11:6
Which statement is true?
Answer: 1, the globus pallidus is lateral to the thalamus.

11:7
Which of the following is not a fold of the dura mater?
Answer: 4, septum pellucidum (this is the thin wall between the two lateral ventricles).

11:8
Which statement about the spinal cord is correct?
Answer: 3, the dorsal root ganglia lie outside of the spinal cord. The ventral and dorsal roots join and form the spinal nerves, the dorsal roots carry afferent signals, and the grey matter occasionally bulges and forms lateral horns.

11:9
Which statement is correct?
Answer: 2, visual signals from the lateral part of the right retina pass the right thalamus (signals from the medial part of the retina cross over, reach the thalamus after the optic chiasma, and leave the thalamus in the optic radiation, not the optic tract).

11:10
Which structure connects the third and fourth ventricles?
Answer: 1, aqueduct of Sylvius.

Questions 111-120

12:1
Which part of the ventricular system lies between the cerebellum and the pons?
1: Lateral ventricle
2: Third ventricle
3: Aqueduct
4: Fourth ventricle
5: Central canal

12:2
The cerebrospinal fluid within the ventricular system is in continuity with which space?
1: Epidural space
2: Extracranial space
3: Subarachnoid space
4: Subdural space

12:3
What is the dorsal part of the mesencephalon known as?
1: Obex
2: Tectum
3: Tegmentum
4: Tonsil

12:4
Which statement about the dorsal columns of the spinal cord is correct?
1: Ascending tract, fibers decussate in the medulla oblongata
2: Ascending tract, fibers decussate in the spinal cord
3: Descending tract, fibers decussate in the medulla oblongata
4: Descending tract, fibers decussate in the spinal cord

12:5
Which structure is found at the tip of the inferior tail of the caudate nucleus?
1: Amygdala
2: Fornix
3: Obex
4: Putamen

12:6
Which structure is found in the Turkish saddle (the sella turcica)?
1: Hypophysis
2: Hypothalamus
3: Mammillary body
4: Pineal gland

12:7
Which term best describes the position of the crista galli in relation to the clivus?
1: Anterior
2: Lateral
3: Medial
4: Posterior

12:8
Which numbers correspond to the glossopharyngeal, accessory and abducens nerve?
1: IX, XI and VI
2: XI, XII and VII
3: VI, VII and IX
4: IX, X and V
5: VII, XI and X

12:9
What lies immediately anterior to the postcentral gyrus of the cerebrum?
1: Central sulcus
2: Postcentral sulcus
3: Precentral gyrus
4: Precentral sulcus

12:10
Which structures would blood from the superior cerebral veins normally pass in their journey to the internal jugular vein, and in which order?
1: Basal vein
2: Confluence of sinuses
3: Great cerebral vein
4: Inferior sagittal sinus
5: Occipital sinus
6: Sigmoid sinus
7: Straight sinus
8: Superior sagittal sinus
9: Transverse sinus

Answers 111-120

12:1
Which part of the ventricular system lies between the cerebellum and the pons?
Answer: 4, fourth ventricle.

12:2
The cerebrospinal fluid within the ventricular system is in continuity with which space?
Answer: 3, subarachnoid space.

12:3
What is the dorsal part of the mesencephalon known as?
Answer: 2, tectum.

12:4
Which statement about the dorsal columns of the spinal cord is correct?
Answer: 1, Ascending tract, fibers decussate in the medulla oblongata.

12:5
Which structure is found at the tip of the inferior tail of the caudate nucleus?
Answer: 1, amygdala.

12:6
Which structure is found in the Turkish saddle (the sella turcica)?
Answer: 1, hypophysis.

12:7
Which term best describes the position of the crista galli in relation to the clivus?
Answer: 1, anterior.

12:8
Which numbers correspond to the glossopharyngeal, accessory and abducens nerve?
Answer: 1, IX, XI and VI (V is the trigeminal nerve, XII is the hypoglossal nerve, VII is the facial nerve, and X is the vagus nerve).

12:9
What lies immediately anterior to the postcentral gyrus of the cerebrum?
Answer: 1, central sulcus.

12:10
Which structures would blood from the superior cerebral veins normally pass in their journey to the internal jugular vein, and in which order?
Answer: 8, 2, 9 and 6, superior sagittal sinus, confluence of sinuses, transverse sinus, and sigmoid sinus.

Questions 121-130

13:1
Which nucleus is found dorsal and medial to the substantia nigra in the mesencephalon?
1: Dentate nucleus
2: Locus coeruleus
3: Nucleus ambiguus
4: Red nucleus

13:2
Moving backwards from the internal jugular vein to the basal vein (vein of Rosenthal), which structures would you normally pass? And in which order?
1: Cavernous sinus
2: Confluence of sinuses
3: Great cerebral vein
4: Inferior sagittal sinus
5: Occipital sinus
6: Sigmoid sinus
7: Straight sinus
8: Superior sagittal sinus
9: Transverse sinus

13:3
In an axial section of the spinal cord, the grey matter has two points pointing backwards and two points pointing forwards. What are they called?
1: Dorsal and ventral horns
2: Superior and inferior horns
3: Dorsal and ventral roots
4: Superior and inferior roots

13:4
Which cranial nerve innervates the muscles involved in mastication?

1: Facial nerve
2: Glossopharyngeal nerve
3: Hypoglossal nerve
4: Trigeminal nerve

13:5
From which part of the lateral ventricles do the interventricular foramina extend?
1: Anterior horn
2: Body
3: Inferior horn
4: Posterior horn

13:6
What is true about the dentate nucleus?
1: It is the smallest of the deep cerebellar nuclei
2: It is the most lateral of the four deep cerebellar nuclei
3: It is rarely visible in a section
4: It is sometimes grouped together with the emboliform nucleus and called the interposed nucleus

13:7
The extreme capsule runs between which two structures?
1: Thalamus and globus pallidus
2: Globus pallidus and putamen
3: Putamen and claustrum
4: Claustrum and insula

13:8
Which two structures do not pass the foramen magnum?
1: Internal carotid arteries
2: Vertebral arteries
3: Spinal cord
4: Accessory nerve (cranial part)
5: Accessory nerve (spinal part)

13:9

What is true about the supratentorial compartment?

1: It refers to all of the structures of the nervous system found above the foramen magnum

2: It refers to all of the structures of the nervous system found below the foramen magnum

3: It refers to all of the structures of the nervous system found above the tentorium cerebelli

4: It refers to all of the structures of the nervous system found below the tentorium cerebelli

13:10

Where in the cerebrum do you find the lingual gyrus?

1: Frontal lobe

2: Occipital lobe

3: Parietal lobe

4: Temporal lobe

Answers 121-130

13:1
Which nucleus is found dorsal and medial to the substantia nigra in the mesencephalon?
Answer: 4, red nucleus.

13:2
Moving backwards from the internal jugular vein to the basal vein (vein of Rosenthal), which structures would you normally pass? And in which order?
Answer: 6, 9, 2, 7 and 3, sigmoid sinus, transverse sinus, confluence of sinuses, straight sinus and great cerebral vein.

13:3
In an axial section of the spinal cord, the grey matter has two points pointing backwards and two points pointing forwards. What are they called?
Answer: 1, dorsal and ventral horns (note, however, that posterior, anterior and column sometimes are used instead of dorsal, ventral and horn, respectively).

13:4
Which cranial nerve innervates the muscles involved in mastication?
Answer: 4, trigeminal nerve.

13:5
From which part of the lateral ventricles do the interventricular foramina extend?
Answer: 1, anterior horn.

13:6
What is true about the dentate nucleus?
Answer: 2, it is the most lateral of the four deep cerebellar nuclei.

13:7
The extreme capsule runs between which two structures?
Answer: 4, claustrum and insula.

13:8
Which two structures do not pass the foramen magnum?
Answer: 1 and 4, the internal carotid arteries and the cranial part of the accessory nerve.

13:9
What is true about the supratentorial compartment?
Answer: 3, it refers to all of the structures of the nervous system found above the tentorium cerebelli.

13:10
Where in the cerebrum do you find the lingual gyrus?
Answer: 2, occipital lobe.

Questions 131-140

14:1
Where do you find the cerebral peduncle?
1: Cerebellum
2: Medulla oblongata
3: Mesencephalon
4: Pons

14:2
Two of these alternatives are nuclei found in the deep white matter of the cerebellum. Which two?
1: Ambiguus
2: Fastigial
3: Flocculus
4: Globose
5: Vermis

14:3
Which structures are found immediately lateral to the third ventricle?
1: Inferior colliculi
2: Putamen
3: Superior colliculi
4: Thalamus

14:4
Which structures and in which order would a motor signal from the frontal lobe travel through?
1: Contralateral internal capsule
2: Contralateral lateral corticospinal tract
3: Contralateral spinothalamic tract
4: Ipsilateral internal capsule
5: Ipsilateral lateral corticospinal tract
6: Ipsilateral spinothalamic tract

14:5

If you are at a point in the parietal lobe and move rostrally, where would you end up?
1: Frontal lobe
2: Mesencephalon
3: Occipital lobe
4: Temporal lobe

14:6

Which artery serves the superior parts of the temporal
lobes?
1: Anterior cerebral artery
2: Middle cerebral artery
3: Posterior cerebral artery
4: Basilar artery

14:7

In a sagittal section, the corpus callosum points forward
(A) and then becomes thinner as it turns down and to the
back (B). What are the names of structures A and B?
1: Genu and rostrum
2: Genu and splenium
3: Rostrum and genu
4: Rostrum and splenium
5: Splenium and genu
6: Splenium and rostrum

14:8

What lies immediately posterior to the precentral sulcus
of the cerebrum?
1: Central sulcus
2: Postcentral gyrus
3: Postcentral sulcus
4: Precentral gyrus

14:9
What is also traveling through the optic canal together
with the optic nerve?
1: Oculomotor nerve
2: Trochlear nerve
3: Abducens nerve
4: Ophthalmic artery
5: Ophthalmic veins

14:10
Which two statements are true about the second branch
(V2) of the trigeminal nerve?
1: It leaves the cranium through the foramen ovale
2: It leaves the cranium through the superior orbital fissure
3: It is the maxillary branch
4: It handles sensory information from the lower eyelid
5: It transmits taste signals from the anterior two-thirds of
the tongue
6: It transmits taste signals from the posterior one-third of
the tongue

Answers 131-140

14:1
Where do you find the cerebral peduncle?
Answer: 3, mesencephalon.

14:2
Two of these alternatives are nuclei found in the deep white matter of the cerebellum. Which two?
Answer: 2 and 4, fastigial and globose.

14:3
Which structures are found immediately lateral to the third ventricle?
Answer: 4, the left and right thalamus.

14:4
Which structures and in which order would a motor signal from the frontal lobe travel through?
Answer: 4 and 2, ipsilateral internal capsule and con-tralateral lateral spinothalamic tract.

14:5
If you are at a point in the parietal lobe and move ros-trally, where would you end up?
Answer: 1, frontal lobe.

14:6
Which artery serves the superior parts of the temporal lobes?
Answer: 2, middle cerebral artery.

14:7
In a sagittal section, the corpus callosum points forward (A) and then becomes thinner as it turns down and to the back (B). What are the names of structures A and B?
Answer: 1, genu and rostrum.

14:8
What lies immediately posterior to the precentral sulcus of the cerebrum?
Answer: 4, precentral gyrus.

14:9
What is also traveling through the optic canal together with the optic nerve?
Answer: Ophthalmic artery (the other structures mentioned use the superior orbital fissure, although branches of the ophthalmic veins use other routes).

14:10
Which two statements are true about the second branch (V2) of the trigeminal nerve?
Answer: 3 and 4, it is the maxillary branch and it handles sensory information from the lower eyelid.

Questions 141-150

15:1
What runs in the internal acoustic meatus?
1: Cochlear nerve only
2: Vestibular nerve only
3: Vestibulocochlear nerve only
4: Vestibulocochlear nerve and facial nerve

15:2
Which artery serves the inferior parts of the temporal lobes?
1: Anterior cerebral artery
2: Middle cerebral artery
3: Posterior cerebral artery
4: Basilar artery

15:3
Which term best describes the position of the sella turcica in relation to the cauda equina?
1: Caudal
2: Lateral
3: Medial
4: Rostral

15:4
Which of the cranial bones are connected by the coronal suture?
1: Ethmoid bone
2: Frontal bone
3: Occipital bone
4: Parietal bone
5: Sphenoid bone
6: Temporal bone

15:5
Which statement is true about the cerebellum?
1: The flocculonodular lobe is found between the anterior and posterior lobes
2: The horizontal fissure separates the anterior lobe from the posterior lobe
3: The horizontal fissure separates the posterior lobe from the flocculonodular lobe
4: The cerebellum is found in the posterior cranial fossa

15:6
Which statement is true?
1: The thalamus is medial to the third ventricle
2: The extreme capsule is medial to the external capsule
3: The external capsule is medial to the claustrum
4: The lentiform nucleus is medial to the internal capsule

15:7
Moving from a lateral ventricle to the central canal, which structures do you pass, and in what order?
1: Aqueduct, third ventricle, interventricular foramen, fourth ventricle
2: Aqueduct, third ventricle, median aperture, fourth ventricle
3: Interventricular foramen, third ventricle, aqueduct, fourth ventricle
4: Interventricular foramen, third ventricle, median aperture, fourth ventricle
5: Median aperture, third ventricle, aqueduct, fourth ventricle
6: Median aperture, third ventricle, interventricular foramen, fourth ventricle

15:8
Where in the brainstem are the oculomotor (CN III) and trochlear (CN IV) nuclei found?
1: Both are in the mesencephalon
2: Both are in the pons
3: CN III in the mesencephalon, CN IV in the pons
4: CN IV in the mesencephalon, CN III in the pons

15:9
Which two statements are true about the spinocerebellar tracts?
1: They are ascending tracts
2: They are descending tracts
3: They run contralateral to the source of the sensory signal
4: They run ipsilateral to the source of the sensory signal

15:10
Where in the cerebrum do you find the straight gyrus?
1: Frontal lobe
2: Occipital lobe
3: Parietal lobe
4: Temporal lobe

Answers 141-150

15:1
What runs in the internal acoustic meatus?
Answer: 4, vestibulocochlear nerve and facial nerve.

15:2
Which artery serves the inferior parts of the temporal lobes?
Answer: 3, posterior cerebral artery.

15:3
Which term best describes the position of the sella turcica in relation to the cauda equina?
Answer: 4, rostral.

15:4
Which of the cranial bones are connected by the coronal suture?
Answer: 2 and 4, the frontal and parietal bones.

15:5
Which statement is true about the cerebellum?
Answer: 4, the cerebellum is found in the posterior cranial fossa.

15:6
Which statement is true?
Answer: 3, the external capsule is medial to the claustrum.

15:7
Moving from a lateral ventricle to the central canal, which structures do you pass, and in what order?
Answer: 3, interventricular foramen, third ventricle, aqueduct, fourth ventricle

15:8
Where in the brainstem are the oculomotor (CN III) and trochlear (CN IV) nuclei found?
Answer: 1, both are in the mesencephalon.

15:9
Which two statements are true about the spinocerebellar tracts?
Answer: 1 and 4, they are ascending tracts that run ipsi-lateral to the source of the sensory signal.

15:10
Where in the cerebrum do you find the straight gyrus?
Answer: 1, frontal lobe.

Thank you!

Thank you for reading this introduction to neuroanatomy! I hope that you will find it useful during your studying.

If you find any kind of error or mistake in the text or in the questions, or if you want to join an e-mail list to receive notifications whenever there is something new coming out, my e-mail address is:

magnusbergmanmd@gmail.com

Sources

A text such as this one is not based on only one or a few sources. It is the result of an accumulation of information from lectures, notes and book studies during medical school, teachings from senior colleagues during clinical rotations, practical knowledge obtained during internship and residency, and bits and pieces hunted down every now and then when needed. It is therefore not possible to assign a reference to every piece of information mentioned here.

However, from time to time during the writing I have consulted three sources that have been very valuable, and if you are unsure about which books to buy in order to continue and deepen your neuroanatomy studies, these are highly recommended. These books are:

Mancall, Elliott L, David G Brock. *Gray's Clinical Neuroanatomy: The Anatomic Basis for Clinical Neuroscience*. Philadelphia: Elsevier Saunders, 2011. Web.

Mtui, Estomih, Gregory Gruener and Peter Dockery. *Fitzgerald's Clinical Neuroanatomy and Neuroscience*. 7th ed. Oxford: Elsevier, 2016. Web.

Vanderah, Todd W. *Nolte's Essentials of the Human Brain*. 2nd ed. Philadelphia: Elsevier, 2019. Web.

Book cover

The image used to create the book cover was downloaded from https://commons.wikimedia.org/wiki/File:Brain_surgery_(1893)_(14781134142).jpg and was uploaded by the user Fae. According to the image's page on Wikimedia Commons, it has "no known copyright restrictions."

*

Made in the USA
Las Vegas, NV
27 September 2024

95872785R10085